HEALTH IN SCHOOLS

Nester Kadzviti Murira

"Children are the future. They need guidance to develop positive attitudes to good health early in life to become health conscious individuals."

Children cannot make decisions on where they can live or who they want to live with. Children cannot make decisions on when to seek health services when they fall ill. Children are therefore a vulnerable group in the community, in a society and in any population in the world because they can be exposed to factors that expose them to ill health.

Children can however master basic health principles and can also inform their parents about what they learn. *"The teacher said this is good for you"* is a statement many parents hear over and over as their children grow; confirming that children can recall information and can be trusted to pass health messages to others.

The above statement also confirms that the teacher has a pivotal role in influencing the quality of life of populations. If children learn to look after their health from an early age, health problems can be reduced and the quality of life of populations can be improved.

This book is written to assist schools in offering health advice to young children, adolescents and college students on fundamental health issues. Each school library should keep a copy of this book and every teacher will find this book a valuable resource. The author is aware that there are differences in infrastructure from one country to another and in urban and rural schools. This book provides a guide line to school health.

Nester Kadzviti Murira

Table of Contents

THE AIM OF THIS BOOK

This book is designed to empower the schoolteacher with health information in selected contemporary health issues that can be shared with the pupils and the community in which the teacher works. Improvement of the health status of the population is the ultimate goal.

This book equips the school teacher with health information and skills to identify ill health among the school children and to take appropriate action accordingly. The book also empowers the school children to become active participants in their personal health issues and preventable health issues in their communities in selected health subjects.

After reading this book, the schoolteacher should be able to:

- Identify abnormal and unhealthy features in a child
- Identify health information needs of school children
- Choose appropriate approaches to providing health information
- Work collaboratively with colleagues or experts in providing health information
- Recognize children's rights
- Advise the school child on basic hygiene
- Advise the school child on healthy eating
- Identify common ailments in school children
- Care for common health ailments
- Provide school children with information on water borne diseases
- Advise the school children on skin diseases
- Identify common neurogenic diseases in the school age child
- Prevent accidents in the school
- Offer appropriate first aid in illness and emergencies in the school
- Advise on matters of puberty, feminine hygiene, HIV/AIDS and substance abuse
- Identify child abuse and take appropriate action
- Offer appropriate health advice to the school leaver

Chapter1

FACTORS THAT INFLUENCE THE HEALTH OF THE CHILD

Children are the future. Healthy children lead to a healthy nation. Children develop good healthy attitudes and behaviours if they are constantly monitored and encouraged to adopt good healthy behaviours. Children learn good health habits from observing good role models.

A child's good health behaviour is a result of combined efforts of responsible adults starting with the child's family. The school teacher is in a very strategic position to identify health problems and to advise the child and his/her family as the one who spends long hours with the child. Health personnel are dependant on decisions made by parents and guardians of the child and usually see the child late after health problems have emerged. Thus the school teacher is the linchpin in promotion of good health in a school age child.

The school teacher therefore is encouraged to liaise with health personnel in planning strategies to promote good health in the school child and planning strategies to prevent health disasters in the school. Through the combined efforts of the family, the school teacher and health personnel, children can be guided to gradually take responsibility of their health at each phase of their development.

Health information and Children

The exposure of children to certain events in their development along the life span improves or deprives the children of good health and appropriate information, attitudes and behaviours to improve their health. Health information specific to the child's stage of development is essential as it enriches children's knowledge of health issues. Health knowledge in children improves children's self care skills, and contributes towards reduction of ill health (morbidity) and unnecessary loss of life (mortality).

As the child grows, he or she is expected to reach and pass through milestones of development that are cumulative adding new dimension in the child's physical, mental, psychosocial and sexual development. These developmental phases are influenced by several factors such as the environment, the diet, access to preventive and curative health care services, the presence or absence of peace, love, prevalence of diseases, as well as cultural practices and expectations.

Children are influenced to a great extent by the environment in which they are brought up. Some environments are ideal and stimulating exposing the child to opportunities to learn and be inquisitive about their health while some environments inhibit the child's development and initiative to explore and learn. The influence of the caregivers or role models plays a major role in what the child learns.

It is therefore crucial that children have access to health information that is age specific and ensures that the child identifies with developmental changes, the body needs and societal expectations at their age. It is important that positive reinforcement in the form of encouragement, positive comments, reminders and repetition are used to assist the child to remember health information and practice good health behaviours always.

The teacher has a very important role in creating health awareness and promoting quality health. The teacher also plays a key role in influencing parents to desist from unfair practices that may lower self -esteem in some children and encourage fairness that includes sharing of chores among children, equal access to basic needs such as food, clothing, shelter and love.

Some cultural practices accepted as the norm in some communities, may impact negatively on the physical and psychosocial health of a child. The teacher can advise the child, the child's parents or guardians and can create health awareness pertaining to the practices as well as alert relevant authorities and groups with special interest on the welfare of the child, on the impact of the practices on the health of the school age child.

Children's Rights

Children have rights just as adults have. Children's rights are human rights. Children's rights can be viewed as needs and opportunities that contribute to making the whole experience of being a child complete and comfortable. The basis of children's rights is the basic human needs.

Psychologist Maslow describes human needs as arranged in a sequence of stratified. It is important that a teacher is familiar with and is reminded of Maslow's hierarchy of human needs. A person has needs or special requirements that one must have to live a fairly comfortable life. These are called physiological needs and are universal cutting across colour, tribe, language and religion. The most important and 'must have' needs are on the lower strata. As the lower levels needs are satisfied, one aspires for higher level needs.

The lowest levels of physiological needs for any human being are those that give life; air to breathe freely, and food. Children have a right and deserve to live where there is free fresh air to breath and access to good food to sustain their lives. Deprivation of food to children is a form of abuse and infringement of children's rights to a decent and comfortable life.

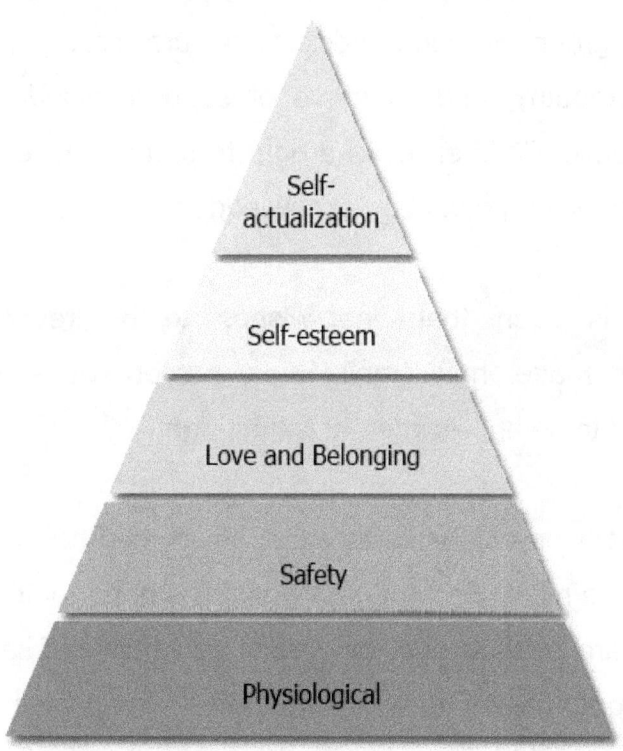

Figure 1 Maslow's Hierarchy of Human Needs (Maslow, 1971)

Maslow's hierarchy of human needs suggests that every human being seeks to fulfil a hierarchy of needs that enables her to survive and feel some satisfaction in life. The needs are illustrated in the above triangle and show the basic and initial needs at the bottom of the triangle. An individual aspires to achieve one level of need before aspiring for a higher level and is not satisfied until she/he attains the highest level of needs, the self actualisation.

When factors that ensure life are in place, an individual will seek safety needs, shelter and protection from wind, rain, unfavourable temperatures. In everyday life one needs decent housing, appropriate clothing and protection from not just the discomforts of the environment but from societal discomforts. Children have a right to decent living and protection against all forms of discomfort, including bullying, exposure to cruelty, indecency and anything that frightens them.

Every person wants to belong to a family, various societal groups, and to a specific race among the human race. People want their ethnic groups acknowledged; their countries of origin known, their family trees recognized even their political afiliations known. From these groupings and associations, one derives satisfaction in knowing they are supported and are not alone.

Belonging to a group or some social structure provides one with love, sympathy and empathy, and all forms of support including psychological, social and economic. Children have a right to parental love or guardian love and their desire to belong must be acknowledged.

Human nature is such that one wishes to be recognized for their achievements no matter how small. Every person wants to be respected. Children too want to be appreciated. It is their right.

Finally people want opportunities to excel and show their capabilities to the full and achieve the most. Each person would like opportunities in life in which their aspirations are limitless until they reach a point of self satisfaction or self-actualization. Opportunities for a child to grow psychologically must be made available to enable children to exercise their mental capacity and energies to the maximum.

Deprived Children

Orphaned children and child led families and their problems, have become a common phenomenon in some parts of the world that have been hard hit by the HIV/AIDS pandemic and wars. Loss of parental figures in growing children results in loss of guidance, lowering of living standards such as poor nutritional status, poor attention to general health, destitution that can expose the children to various forms of abuse. The schoolteacher has a role to identify such children at risk and alert respective government ministries and various stakeholders such as well- wishers like religious and charity organizations.

Wars affect the health of populations but the hardest hit are children. In war torn regions, there is general chaos and disorderly displacement of people, destruction of essential facilities and opportunities such as access to adequate health care services. The conflict environment deprives children of a free and normal climate of play, which in itself is an essential component of growing up and learning along the lifeline.

Wars are associated with shortage of food, poor access to fresh adequate drinking water, poor sanitation and its problems such as diarrhoeal diseases. These social, political and environmental problems increase ill health in the population and compromise the health of young people in particular. Teachers working in war torn zones have a challenge to provide children in these areas with general health information to apply the best self care skills possible to prevent ill health and achieve good health despite the difficult times prevailing.

Children must have full immunization and their growth must be regularly monitored to protect them from infectious diseases like poliomyelitis, tuberculosis, measles and whooping cough. The teacher has an important role to liaise with parents and health authorities to ensure that all children have been vaccinated against preventable diseases where possible. Close monitoring of health records prevents and ensures that all children have regular health checks to prevent the likelihood of epidemics of preventable diseases in schools.

Children must be closely monitored for nutritional diseases that affect physical growth and predispose them to ill health.

Child labour is exposing children to hard work meant for adults such as farm work, mining and other industries as well as domestic work in homes. Child labour deprives children and robs them of an opportunity to grow and enjoy the stages of their childhood as well as achieve full potential of their development. Teachers have a role to identify such disadvantaged children and initiate discussions with parent and social services to assist children in deprived environments to enjoy their rights to be children.

Family instability such as separation of parents and divorce may push children into unsuitable arrangements in which there may not be commitment, enthusiasm and means to provide basics like food, love and guidance required for healthy growth of children. Family instability compromises the growing child's health and may expose the child to physical, mental and sexual abuse.

The teacher is encouraged to identify children who are affected by family wrangles and can initiate a dialogue with relevant authorities like social services and child welfare organizations to attend to the plight of affected children.

References

Maslow, A. (1971). *Motivation and Personality*. New York: Harper & Row.

Chapter 2

THE SCHOOL AGE CHILD

This chapter outlines the normal physical and mental development that enables the school teacher to identify abnormal development in the school child. School age is from the age of five and onwards. A school going child should have marked differences from a toddler.

Physical changes

The school age child shows evidence of growth in height and weight. The child generally has a slimmer outlook with a fair distribution of fat around the body taking over from the babyish chubby looks. The growth rate is steady and boys' and girls' growth rate is alike. Variations without a specific pattern may occur in growth spurts until the age of twelve. Long bones grow considerably and continue to do so into adolescence, and so do other parts of the body.

Muscle mass increases along with strength especially with boys who are slightly stronger than girls although this difference may only be significant around puberty. The child has loads of energy that seem to increase by the day. There are of course exceptions to the rule that may deliberately sit back and are reluctant to participate in activity. A child who is inactive should draw a teacher's attention and curiosity to find out why the child behaves that way.

Skills

The child has developed the basic motor skills like dressing, brushing teeth, lacing up shoes and can wash herself although help may be needed in this task. Children are keen to display newly found skills and will repeatedly perform these. The child's nervous system is fairly well developed and allows more control and coordination of tasks. A child who struggles with basic tasks such as lacing up shoes, for example, removing a cardigan when hot or wearing it may need to be observed to enable a feedback to health authorities or to parents.

Nerve development, bone and muscular changes combine to increase the child's abilities.

Mental Abilities

There is considerable brain growth between 7-8years of age increasing the brain function and the capacity to think. The child can tell a coherent short story, is capable of reading, counting and writing although these skills are still at their rudimentary stage. Most body systems reach their maturity during this stage of development. Development of competences is based on and influenced by family supervision and encouragement and association with peers.

The environment in which the child grows is a key factor in the child's development. A stimulating environment increases curiosity and development of more advanced and intricate skills. A child who is allowed freedom to perform tasks under supervision develops confidence and skills faster than the child whose parents are over protective.

The Skin

Hair darkens and adopts its final color at this stage of development. The skin is slowly adopting an adult appearance. The sweat glands and other skin glands are almost inactive. A child can play and run up and down without any sweat on the face or body.

The Immune System

The school age is the healthiest span of life in an individual. The child has almost completed her/his immunization schedule and immunity in the body should now be fully established as a result, children have quick recovery from illness. The child has high levels of energy which exposes him/her to accidents like falls, cuts, and bruises. Injuries heal fast because the child has high levels of immunity.

The Gastro-Intestinal (GIT) System

The maturity of the GIT system is seen by the ability of the child to eat and tolerate adult foods. The child's appetite is good and the child wants to eat frequently. It is important to encourage children to eat well, a balanced diet with a lot of fruit and vegetables and to emphasize on the healthy eating avoiding junk oily food that may lead to child obesity. Some children may develop health complications like breathing problems, kidney problems and heart problems due to overweight. Lack of nutritious foods in adequate amounts may lead to undernourishment.

The teacher may advise on contents of healthy snacks that a child may bring to school. A balanced snack would be composed of all food groups and especially green vegetables, fruit, and energy foods.

Health Advice

A child must have three full meals per day and nutritious snacks, fruit, fruit juices or milk in between meals. It is important that parents are advised to prepare nutritious well balanced snacks for children to eat at school. Parents should be advised especially where a child shows signs of poor diet to have at least one major meal with the child in order for the parents to observe the child's pattern of eating and encourage the child to eat well. Where there is a school health system in place, teachers can forward such children's names to the school nurse. Almost all the systems mature during this stage **except for the reproductive system**, which does not develop fully until puberty.

Respiratory System

The lungs mature and the child can now take in deep inspiration and expiration breaths and considerable amount of air is moved in and out of the lungs increasing lung expansion as the child runs around and plays. Respirations become slower, and range between 17-25 per minute. If a child breathes faster than this rate, this is a sign of respiratory distress and that the lungs are not fully expanding and taking in enough air. Respiratory distress is common in such conditions like asthma, pneumonia and other lung diseases and also in high fevers. The child with respiratory distress must be quickly referred to a health centre, doctor or hospital for health tests, treatment and advice.

The Circulatory System

The heart increases in size but the heart rate slows down to an average of 72 beats per minute. To check for the heart beat (pulse) fingers are held firmly but not tightly against the bone of the lower arm just after the wrist, or fingers are placed flat on the head between the ear and the eyes, the temporal region. High fevers and loss of body fluid such as in diarrhoea and vomiting, and haemorrhage may cause the heart to beat faster.

Health Advice

Children must have a yearly health check. It is important that there is a school health system that enables health personnel to check each child's health yearly. Records of the child should be kept to monitor the health of the child.

Lymphatic System

The body protection system or the lymphatic system develops considerably and there is increase of lymphoid tissue marked by large tonsils. Tonsils are part of the body protection mechanisms that fight infections particularly such infections that are likely to get into the body through the respiratory system and through the mouth.

Sex differences

Girls' permanent teeth erupt sooner than boys.
Girls mature and grow much faster than boys.

Race Difference

Black and Asian children mature faster than white children. This is thought to be related to genes, upbringing and cultural expectations, socio-economic factors and dietary factors (Edelman & Mandle, 1995).

Genetic Influence

Genes from both parents genetically influence the child's rate of growth and the height but diet makes a lot of difference to children's growth.

Elimination

Full bowel and bladder control should be established by six years. A child getting adequate fluids should empty her bladder at least six to eight times per day. A child should empty her bowels at least once or twice a day.

Enuresis

Enuresis is poor bladder control. Enuresis can be due to a reduced bladder capacity. Loss of bladder control is associated with stress at home and some environmental factors such as unfamiliar or threatening surroundings. It may be necessary to discuss with parents or refer the child to a child psychologist. Enuresis is also associated with genetic predisposition and delay in nerve development responsible for bladder contraction reflex. This slows down the child's response to a full bladder. Infections such as urinary tract infection may interfere with bladder control. The child often develops low self-esteem and poor self- confidence.

It is important to discourage peers from teasing the child. Encouraging children to empty the bladder at regular intervals such as two to four hourly may help children with bladder control problems to get control of their bladders. The child should be referred to health personnel to exclude underlying health problems. Parents should be advised against becoming too hard on the child before thorough investigations are done. The parents can be referred to health personnel for more information, support and encouragement in dealing with the problem.

Poor control of the bowel

The boy child may have poor control of the bowel in emotional difficulties. The child may complain of abdominal pain or may have no complaints at all. It may be necessary to discuss with the child and his family and agree to establish a special bowel-emptying programme. Health personnel may be called upon to provide counselling to both parents and child

Cognition and Perceptual Development

Development of basic senses, language, skills and memory should improve as the child grows.

Between the age of 7-11years the child consolidates on his/her skills and learns to master many skills possible.

The child moves from egocentric thinking and behaviour to cooperative interactions where she no longer takes a centre stage but realises the presence of others and importance of including others and is prepared to share. There are however a few who will remain egocentric and selfish who may need patience and persuasion to realise that there are other people around them.

Mentally, the child gradually develops the capacity to answer to questions in sentences and not one word (monologue). This makes conversation possible as the child can relate events and can tell stories. The child also shows signs of ability to reason and does not act out of intuition but stops to think. The child displays **logic** like arranging things in an order. The child can add and subtract. The child is able to classify things according to relationships and characteristics e.g. birds, animals, and his/her various play toys.

The child can perceive things that she can see. The ability to perceive abstract things is not yet developed at this stage. This is why the child needs to see pictures in a story book to remember the story; and needs to see beads, pebbles, marbles, oranges, or any items to count them and subtract them. As the child continues to grow, the child thinks differently from the pre-school child and listens to others' views.

The child develops the concept of time and does not want to be delayed for activities of importance to her like school or parties.

Vision

The child has developed the optimum visual capacity by the age of 7years. He/she should be able to discriminate fine differences and similarities if given two or more almost similar pictures or items. However not all children have perfect eyesight. At least 20% of children at this age may have visual problems some of which are obvious and some which can only be detected on examination by health personnel.

Common visual problems

Near-sightedness or myopia is difficulty in seeing objects that are far. This condition is caused by an elongated eyeball. The child will not be able to read what is at the front of the classroom when seated in the back row. Some children may improve dramatically once they change the sitting angle. It is however important to refer a child with such a problem to health personnel for thorough eye tests and correction of sight problems.

Far-sightedness or Hyperopia is difficulty in seeing objects that are close by. A child ho has problems seeing things that are close by benefit by change of position and eyesight correction by health personnel.

Astigmatism or squint, is poor focus on images.
Blurred vision is a lack of clarity of shape, colors and details of what is seen. A child with such problems should be referred to an optician who may decide to correct the problem by special glasses or refer the child to an eye surgeon for some minor surgical procedure to correct the eye focus.

Hearing

The child's hearing ability or accuracy should be very sharp by the age of 7years. Hearing problems are however less common than visual problems and are usually caused by mild inflammation or fluid in the middle ear.

All school age children should have annual hearing evaluations done by health personnel.

By late childhood, children have learnt to combine visual, auditory and tactile senses to interpret and understand the world around them. For some children one of the senses may be more developed than the other. It is important to appreciate that no two children have the same sensory acuity. This is what makes them have different perceptions and conceptions of the world around them.

Discrimination of details may come later on as the child continues to grow for instance some children may have difficulty in differentiating d and b, a and o, l and r, and 6and 9 as well as w and m. It is important to exercise patience with such children considering that child development does not occur at the same rate and only refer them for assessment where the perception is really poor.

Language development

Children have the ability to understand and speak a language commonly spoken around them. The capacity to learn a second language is at its maximum around seven years of age, especially where children live in an environment encouraging learning two languages. The child should be able to articulate all sounds in languages although s, l, and r, can be the problem letters. A six year old should have a spoken vocabulary of at least 2000 words.

Children learn differently though. Some learn by sounding out each single word (phonetics), while others aim at learning the whole word as a chunk or a combination of both.

In reading, conceptual, perceptual and verbal skills are used. This is what makes reading difficult for most children. Many skills included in the development of language e.g. visual perception, reading, auditory acuity, and perception to understand spoken language are present by the age of seven so are fine motor skills for articulation and handwriting. It is therefore important to expose children to as much reading material as possible to improve language, the skills to read and perceive concepts. This can be made easy by exposing children to the library early in their learning from pre-school where such facilities exist. Parents should be encouraged to acquire books and any reading materials for their children.

Where libraries are not available such as in poor country communities, it is possible to appeal for and collect old books from old pupils, appeal to local government and education ministries and to well wishers for book donations to start a small collection of books for the children. Parents can be encouraged to make as much contribution as possible.

By the time the child is about eight or nine, he/she understands grammar, meanings, and understands multiple meanings of the same words. At this age a child should be able to recognize spelling and grammar errors.

Handwriting

Writing requires hand- eye coordination, nerve control of muscle and joints as well as perceptual abilities. Handwriting is a skill and does not need intelligence. Like any skill, a child needs repeated practice, to gradually learn to shape letters and improve hand writing. Boys have more problems in writing legibly than girls.

Some children are more comfortable writing with their right hand while others prefer the left hand. If a child prefers to use one hand, they should not be discouraged.

Both short term and long term memory improve for the school age child
A child can use learning strategies like organizing, classifying, labelling, rehearsal and repetition to help her remember learning material.

Intelligence

Intelligence is the quantity of ability to think a person has compared to others. There are intelligence test scores that are used to test how intelligent an individual is. This is only necessary where a child shows' learning difficulty and it becomes necessary to conduct tests to identify the amount of deficit the child has and to plan for the appropriate assistance the child requires.

Intelligence tests and achievements tests both measure the same thing. Intelligence tests give an **Intelligence Quotient** (IQ) which is the ratio of the individual child's performance compared to others. An IQ of 90-110 is desirable whereas scores below 50 percentile indicate a low IQ. Heredity, deprived environment and poor socio-economic status have a major role to play in influencing intelligence.

Learning Difficulties

Attention Deficit Hyperactivity Disorder (ADHD) This is a condition in a school child characterized by varied degrees of inattention (Edelman & Mandle,1995). The child cannot concentrate on an activity or listen for long periods. The child gets restless and has impulsiveness to do things.
The child is easily distracted by external stimuli. It is important to avoid disruption while this child writes or reads.
A child with ADHD is an impatient person who has difficulty waiting his turn in class or in games. He often blurts out answers to questions before they are completed. He disrupts others as they play. He has difficulty following through instruction therefore has difficulty sustaining attention in tasks or play. He often shifts from one uncompleted activity to another. He often looses things necessary for tasks.

A child with ADHD has difficulty playing quietly and often talks excessively. He interrupts or intrudes on others and does not listen to what is being said to him. The child engages in dangerous activities without considering consequences e.g. jumping from heights, running into a road without checking first.

The schoolteacher must keep an eye on such a child and assist the child as much as possible to fit in the class and participate in activities with little disruption of others.

Minimal Brain Dysfunction

A child may be slow to think, to perceive, or to get involved in activities. Some children are late developers than others. Patience is required with a slow child. It may be ideal to have slow learners in their own class so that they are not discouraged by falling behind fast learners.

Developmental Arithmetic Disorder (DAD)

This is a condition in which a child has difficulty in using numbers (addition, subtraction, division). Patience is required to assist this child and use of counting aids or mathematical aids can help the child improve the ability to count.

Developmental Reading Disorder (DRD)

The child has difficulty in reading, putting together words. the child needs assistance both in class ad at home. Parental participation in helping the child with extra reading, and use of the library may help the child to improve reading skills.

Health Personnel's role

Health personnel play a major role in detection of disability. It is important to work closely with them. Health personnel will help as consultants in seeking specialist services e.g. reference to psychologist and special learning groups. Health personnel will provide support for both parents and child and will arrange for counselling of both child and parents.

Achievements

At the age of 7-11 The child aspires to master tasks to be accomplished. The child is very keen to learn and accomplish both personal and social tasks. The spirit of competitiveness is very high. The child is involved intensely among peers. She shows high levels of interest in what she/he does and concentrates on developing knowledge and skills. Mastery of knowledge and skills is obtained through interaction with peers. The child develops self-concept and wants to be identified through achievements.

The child develops **self-esteem** and believes in herself to be capable of performing tasks and competing with others. She wants to be significant among others through accomplishments and success.

The child's focus is increasingly out of home and with friends. Approval by others is important for development of self-esteem to the child. Peer group influence is significant at this stage of development and there is a tendency to compare achievements of self and of parents. *My father has a big office. Our car is bigger than yours...*

Inferiority

If however the child feels she is not achieving, she may have a sense of inferiority. Repeated failures or poor performance at attempted tasks pulls the child down. The child may loose confidence and becomes withdrawn and full of self-pity. Teacher and family support is important for reassurance, encouragement, and setting firm behaviour guidelines.

Sense of Control

As the child grows, a sense of control over self and environment is developed. The child begins to make choices and feels in charge of herself. Her locus of control is either within her or outside depending on the environment. Children with an internal locus of control are achievers and determined to do better all the time.

The child feels she is responsible for her behaviour and accomplishments. Some children however may not be forth coming, often waiting for a push or command from the teacher to get involved or work harder. They need patience and encouragement to bring out their best performance and to give them a competitive spirit.

Depression and Stress

There are many stressors that may affect the normal development of a child such as change of environment, change of school, change of teacher, stiff competition, failure, family discord, loss of a parent, living with foster parents, having rigid parents and having physical deformity.

Stress may bring about a state of anxiety and helplessness in which a child may fail to cope with the stress and may transfer the stress to a physical problem (somatisation), where a child may complain of headache, stomach ache or pain in any part of the body. This kind of pain is often referred to as functional or psychogenic pain. Children may develop discrete repetitive movement such as clicking finger joints repeatedly, or moving any part of the body repeatedly. Such habits are called *tics,* a manifestation of anxiety or tension in the child. Should such behaviour be observed in a child, discussion with parents or guardian may help to identify the problem or the child may be referred to a psychologist. Depression in a child may affect normal development and functioning.

A depressed child may display the following behaviours, anorexia or loss of appetite, lethargy, aggression, weeping, irritability, frequent day dreaming, low self-esteem. The child may display school refusal learning problems and loss of interest in previously enjoyed activities. The teacher should be patient with such a child and encourage the child to disclose the source of her worries.

Moral Behavior

The child 's judgement of moral behaviours may initially be unclear and goes through several stages of refinement as the child grows. The child's judgments are the ability to figure out if something is right or wrong. The child's behaviour and feelings are greatly influenced by the environment at home, at school, within the society and are based on role models within those institutions.

The stage of moral judgments in the school age child is controversial because it could be that children avoid doing certain things because they are afraid to be punished, and not necessarily that they have developed moral judgment. Moral development however develops in four stages, namely:

Stage 1. Punishment and obedience. The child may not do certain things because he knows he will be punished and will display behaviours that enable him to get favours form parents or guardian.

Stage 2   Individualism, instrumental purpose, and exchange. The child may be ego-centric but will comply with rules in exchange for gains.

Stage 3.   Good boy versus bad boy

A child will behave well for the praises he gets. If he is continuously praised for good behavior he will behave well to enjoy the praise.

Stage 4.   Law and order

Many children are at stage 2 by the time they go to school. In later childhood, children progress to the conventional level, which includes stages 3 and 4.

In the conventional stage, the child looks at others and the laws of institutions and society at large for approval of actions and definition of rules.

This stage coincides with Piaget's cognitive level of concrete operations and the child's increased interaction with the outside world (Edelman & Mandle, 1995).

Moral Behaviour Problems

Some moral behaviour problems that are common during the school age are, **lying, stealing**, and **cheating**. Children may lie because they are afraid of being punished.

Children cheat because of a desire to win or do well.

Children steal when they think they will not be caught and if they think that it is the only way for them to get what they want. These behaviours must be discouraged because if a child knows that he/she can get away with lying, theft and cheating, he/she will probably repeat these behaviours until they become a habit. Parents need reassurance that these are common developmental behaviours and that the child is normal but that they have to play their role in discouraging such behaviour.

Health Perception

The school age child is old enough to understand some health concepts and principles and some behaviours that may cause ill health.

Most children may have learnt some preventive health practices from parents and peers such as brushing teeth, washing hands, eating well. It should not however be taken for granted that all children have this information.

Depending on the communities one is dealing with, some children may be hearing these health practices for the first time. An assessment of the child's perceptions of health is important before teaching them health issues.

All children will need reinforcements on healthy behaviours. It is important that children need to understand the causes of illness and the preventive measures. This information gives the child a strong foundation of the principles of health. It is important to tell children the truth about the causes of illness to reduce misconceptions. Parents too should be encouraged to tell children as much as they can. Children too are very good health promoters because they can be trusted to carry health messages to their parents and their peers.

It is important to give children an opportunity to ask questions about their health to get more information that helps them to develop self—care skills early in life.

Relationships

Parents and children interact in a variety of ways. There is usually attachment, love, companionship that exists between them. During the school age the relationship may shift as the child begins to develop independence and picking her own friends.

Relationships with siblings vary according to sex and ages of the children. Siblings play an important role as playmates, and the child may practice teacher-learner, protector-dependent roles with her siblings. Rivalry may also occur. This is expected in the process of growing up fortunately for the school age child, friends outside the home limit rivalry with siblings.

Both parents and teachers have a role in limit setting to teach the child behaviours that are acceptable in the society. A child needs clear limits and parental and teacher expectations to make it easier for the child to comply and learn what is acceptable. Children model their behaviour according to what they see. Positive reinforcement is important in a child's development.

Community Relationships

Children develop strong relationships with their peers. Peers act as a new social system and become increasingly influential in a child's life. Children learn values, behaviors and attitudes from their peers and parents. Friendships that develop at entry into school and in early years in school may change by age 9-10 years and on leaving primary school. This change is brought about by re-identification of aspirations and attitudes. Children will continue to be influenced by the environment, by family, by culture and by peers. Guidance is important to keep the child under control and with acceptable behavior, values and norms.

References

Edelman, CL & Mandle, CL (1995). Health Promotion Throughout the Lifespan. 4th Edition St. Lewis, MO: Mosby. Galemore.

Chapter 3

HEALTH INFORMATION NEEDS

In some countries, health resources are readily available to children as they grow up. There are clearly set health care schedules for children up to school age in some countries while access to health care is limited and does not always reach everyone who needs it in some countries. Through the schools, it is possible to pass on health messages to children and their parents even in the remote parts of a country.

Children may suffer unnecessarily from preventable diseases due to lack of basic knowledge of health in those with the responsibility to care for them. Some children get to the health facilities so late that what may have started off as a minor health problem has become complicated to the extent of crippling the life of the child.

A teacher is a role model not only for the learners, but also to the community at large. Children accept unreservedly what they are told by their teachers and strive to emulate their teachers in many ways. Children look up to the teacher for guidance and expect the teacher *to act what he says*. Through the teacher, children can learn how to keep healthy and to guard against ill health.

The teacher uses his/her influence on the children to improve their health and help them acquire new information in health and the **teacher is therefore a health model**. The pupils understand health issues better and find it easy to follow advice on health issues if they readily see good examples around them.

Individuals, families and communities have health information needs that may be unique to them. The need for health information may arise as a result of prevailing health problems within the community one lives in, or because one has need for information on a special problem she/he or a close relative may have.

Health information is empowering as it enables one to understand their health better (Ewles &Simnet,1999). Schools can play a major role in equipping children with self-care skills to manage their health and promote good health and enjoy quality life.

Assessing health information needs

A few questions can be posed to help identify health information needs as follows:

Is there a health information need?

Who says there is a need?

Who needs the information?

What kind of information is needed?

What is the source of the information?

How can the information be given?

There are indicators to an information deficit, which may appear as

- Unhealthy behaviours displayed by pupils
- An outbreak of preventable diseases
- Unfounded rumours or societal beliefs

Who says there is need for information?

- The teacher can identify the need for information through observation of unhealthy practises, by asking questions or may hear untrue health statements
- The pupils can ask for information
- Members of the community, the parents can ask for information about a health problem
- The state may indicate the need for specific information

Who needs the information?

Before health information can be given, it is important that it is clear who is to benefit from the information, *the target person/group/population.* This is important to enable appropriate messages to be sent to the right people in the right amounts and appropriate language. Information can be for the following people:

- The pupils in general or in special groups like boys, or girls; special ages like below seven or teenagers
- The parents may need information as a group or it could be specific information required by one parent
- The teacher(s) may need information to help them cope with a specific problem noticed in the school.

What kind of information is needed?

It is important to verify the nature of the health information needs.

Individual interviews or group interviews can be used to find out the needs of a target group.

Observation of the group or individual may reveal information need.

Types of information needs

Felt needs" and *"expressed needs*" The prospective learners will express the type of information that they are keen to acquire; that which matters to them most.

Pressing needs or **the urgent needs** according to the target population should then be identified and attended to first. What will be learnt will capture the group's interest if it responds to the group's concerns. This will probably be information responding to the challenges the group is currently facing.

Normative needs are based on the set standards in the syllabus. These may not necessarily focus on what the learners want to know but will fulfil a requirement set by curriculum planners.

Comparative needs are information requests that the learners are bringing forward because another class or another school has access to the information. The learners are comparing themselves to another group or another class. The standards of information that a school may aspire to achieve may be similar to those enjoyed elsewhere by a similar group of learners, perhaps in another school or another country.

Levels of health information provision

There are three levels of health information provision that one may choose to use. These are as follows:

Health Information for Primary Prevention

This is information that focuses on:

- Avoidance of harmful habits e.g. Litering attracts rodents, flies and mosquitoes that cause ill health. The children would therefore be advised to keep orderly and avoid littering, habits and practices that attract those disease causing creatures.

- Providing information for positive health behaviour   e.g. Eat fresh fruit and vegetables because they contain vitamins that prevent disease.

Health Promotion

This is information that enables one to uplift one's health and maintain good health.

Example: Eating fruit and vegetables ensure that the body is supplied with vitamins that prevent diseases.

Health promotion also helps the target group to acquire new information.

Example: A child's eyes must be clean and clear and without discharge of any nature. Watery eyes, and pus in the eyes are a sign of eye infection.

Health Education

Health education focuses on a specific health problem. It could be an emergency or a problem affecting one group. **Example:** There is an outbreak of an infectious disease like mumps. The teacher may educate the class about it so that the children know how to prevent its spread, know how to progress, and what to do in case one is infected. Or A child may have mumps and the teacher gives health information and self-care information to the child.

Acquisitions of self- care skills

Information can be given through health education to enable individuals and groups to take an active role to look after themselves.

Example: Feminine hygiene for girls at puberty.

Health information can be **reactive**, that is responding to an already identified need. A reactive programme contains information designed to satisfy identified needs. **Example:** It is discovered that there is a child with head lice. The teacher may give health education to the class on identification, management and prevention of head lice.

Health information can be **proactive**, that is attending to issues that have not yet occurred. This happens when new information that is not known by the target group is given, such as when a new subject is introduced. **Example:** How flies can cause disease. The objectives of the topic have to be clear and where possible, examples from everyday experiences must be quoted to satisfy the learner to appreciate that the material is worth learning.

Approaches to teaching health information

A. Systems Approach

In this approach health issues pertaining to a body system are discussed, e.g. The Circulatory System. The teacher may choose to talk about where blood is formed, the importance of blood to a person, and prevention of blood loss. When talking about The Digestive System, the teacher may want to talk about a balanced diet and how the food is digested and used in the body.

B. Body Parts Approach.

Specific body parts can be singled out and discussed, e.g. the heart, or the ear.

C. ABC's of Health

Health issues can be discussed **alphabetically, e.g.** pertinent health issues that start with the letter "A" like anthrax. When these are exhausted, issues that start with the letter "B" can then be discussed.

D. Selected Subject Areas

This is an approach where health topics are **prioritised** and discussed according to their relevance to the target population.

Example: When talking to children in their first year at school, one may focus on issues like ringworm, scabies, and general body cleanliness. Such topics are more important to that age group than puberty, which may still be years away from this age group.

Choosing an approach

To enable you to choose an appropriate approach to your programme, it is best to go through the following questions:

A. The Target Group

How large is the group?

- *An individual.* The individualized approach is where the individual with a problem is engaged in a conversation on a one to one basis, with the individual expressing her problem, and advice given accordingly, would be ideal.
- A *small group* of boys or girls. Small group approaches such as discussion with each participant taking part in the discussion by expressing his/her opinion would be ideal.
- Is it the *whole school*? Large group approaches like the lecture; a video or slides may be used.

B. What change do you want to see in the target group after the education programme?

- Do you want them to be *just knowledgeable*? This is the *cognitive* level. It is the lowest level of learning. The pupils may acquire information *but may not use it. The danger is the information is easily forgotten.*.

- Do you want them to **change their attitude** to specific aspects of health? This is the second level of learning, the **affective** level.

- Do you want them to **behave differently, make sound health decisions that promote good health**, and do something positive to improve their health, such as being able to persuade others including their families to change? This is the highest level of learning, the **psychomotor** level or the **doing** level.

If you are aiming at the second and third levels, then you need to provide your learners with a source of information such as a handout for reference or involve them in an activity that they will remember for a long time. You will need to devise a way of monitoring progress or mastery of material taught. It is important that you evaluate the success of your programme and be prepared to provide assistance to your learners so that the goals are achieved.

The Learning Programme

- Decide if it consist learning activity and resource materials
- Decide if it will be one or two meetings and distribution of learning materials
- Decide if it will be a series of meetings or a once off exercise

Plan where the resource materials will be **accessed freely**. Is it going to be the notice board or the library? Think of how many pupils will be able to access the material in any particular place you choose.

It may be useful to find out from a local resource centre if they have leaflets and posters that you may use to enhance your educational sessions.

If you have several meetings with your pupils on the subject, then divide your materials into **"manageable chunks"** to enable your learners to assimilate the material. If it is a one off lecture, ensure that your learners have **some notes** or a **handout** to refer to later.

D. The Teacher/Facilitator.

- You may want to work with other teachers
- You may want to invite experts

If you are using Resource Materials Only

- You can collect resource materials for your chosen/identified target group from health facilities and some non -governmental organizations and civic groups who may have ready handouts and leaflets. Decide how much of this material is relevant for the level of learner you are dealing with by going through it before you give it to the learners.
- Decide on what your learners **"must know"**, what is **"nice for them to know"**, and what they **"may know"**.
- Remember that your learners go back to their community. It is important that health information given fosters **"acceptable** *attitudes* **and behaviour"** in the community and does not go against the norms of the society.

Q.E: It is advisable to collect as much information as possible relevant to the topics on your programme in advance, so that should there be conflicting ideas, you have time to consult an expert before the lesson.

Working with colleagues

If you are working with other teachers, plan on what role each one of you will play to provide seamless knowledge and prevent confusion among the learners. You could divide the topic into subheadings and each one of you prepares a subheading and takes turns to share the material with the pupils. Alternatively, you could all prepare learning materials for boys or for girls of a certain age group that you will all share with the pupils in an open forum.

Use of Experts

- Invite a specialist in the subject to your school from your local area (e.g. an environmental health officer, a community health nurse, a dental hygienist, a health promotion officer) to discuss with staff and pupils those topics you are uncomfortable with.

- Ensure that the specialist does not use medical jargon by asking him to clarify issues on behalf of your pupils.
- It is advisable to have in the library some simple medical books that can be used by staff and pupils for reference and also for further explanation of subjects discussed.

Reference

1. Edelman, CL & Mandle, CL (1995). Health Promotion Throughout the Lifespan. 4th Edition St. Lewis, MO: Mosby. Galemore.
2. Ewles, L. and Simnett, I. (1999) Promoting Health. A Practical Guide to Health

Chapter 4

BASIC HYGIENE FOR THE SCHOOL CHILD

The aim of this chapter is to emphasize the principles of cleanliness in the young child, in order to prevent avoidable diseases. Health conscious children will grow up to be health conscious adults. This improves their quality of life. Children come from varying backgrounds with a diversity of health standards and values. The teacher has the task to assist those with low standards of hygiene and health knowledge to raise their standards through encouragement while encouraging those who already have positive health values to keep up their values.

Dressing

While to many people the aim of dressing is just to cover the body, children can be taught to attach certain positive standards to dressing. It should be stressed that one need not have new or good quality clothes to dress well. Good dressing standards can still be achieved with old clothes. Some points that can be emphasized to help children improve the way they dress up are as follows:

- There is need to keep an eye on children's clothes and shoes as they quickly grow out of them. Well fitting clothes allow air to circulate in the body. This enables the body pores to breathe. Children can play freely in well fitting clothes.
- Tight clothes emphasize the ugly curves of the body. They allow sweat to quickly soak into clothes taking away the body freshness. Tight clothes limit a child's ability to move and play freely.
- Torn clothes reflect a picture of an irresponsible and careless person. Children should be encouraged to mend their clothes and replace lost buttons on their clothes to improve their outlook. The old adage, "A stitch in time saves nine" could be emphasized.
- Torn shirt collars carry germs in their fluff. They look untidy. These can be turned or patched by a tailor and look as good as new.

- Children should be encouraged to stitch up loose hems, and torn clothes seams should be mended before they give way.
- Clothes that are creased are untidy and should be discouraged. They can also be a source of germs, lice and skin disease.
- Encourage the pupils to look neat and tidy all the time. This trains them to be responsible individuals and keeps dirt and diseases away.

Repeating Clothes
- Certain clothing items such as knickers and socks should be washed before they can be won again. These clothing items have direct contact with the body sweat and emit an unpleasant odour due to dry sweat on them if they are not washed every time they are worn. This can be very unpleasant to other people close by.
- Children should be encouraged to change their school clothes or wash their school clothes at least twice a week; changing uniforms daily is most ideal. Dirt, dust, and germs collect and stick on children's clothes as they play. Constant washing and ironing removes the dirt and kills germs.

Shoes

Shoes dictate how one walks. Slippers and slops promote shuffling of feet. This raises dust and micro- organisms in the dust which can be carried from one part of the school to the next.
- Worn out heels distort the shape of feet and affect gait. This can be a cause of hip pain and muscular aches and pains in later life. This is also true of high-heeled shoes worn by children. These can be fashionable but they pull muscles, distort the growing hip and spinal bones in young girls and women. This becomes problematic later on in life when hip bones and spinal bones cause discomfort.
- Shoes must be polished daily with shoe polish. This keeps off dust and makes the shoes last longer. Unpolished shoes collect dust that carries germs. Canvas shoes must be washed at least once a week or more often depending on the weather.

- Tight shoes interfere with proper development of feet and legs affecting the child's stature and gait.

Unhygienic Habits

Hands off the Nose

The nose is part of the respiratory system. The nose draws in air and cleans it of dust and micro-organisms before the air is drawn into the lungs to be distributed to the whole body. The nose produces mucus that traps dust and the micro-organisms. This mucus flows out freely carrying with it the dirt it collected.

Ideally nasal discharge must be wiped away, and the nose cleared of the excess mucus. Quite often children may be tempted to wipe their noses with the back of the hand, or worse still draw the mucus back into the nose. This is a bad and unhygienic habit. It draws back micro-organisms that may be a cause for sore throat or lung infection. Sniffing back mucus irritates others and must be strongly discouraged.

Children must be encouraged to have soft facial tissue or a clean handkerchief always to blow the nose of the dirty mucus.

- Children must be discouraged from picking their noses with their fingers. Nails collect the dirty mucus, which can be a source of ill health as fingers handle food.
- Children must be encouraged to blow the nose thoroughly when taking a wash every morning to clear the nose of mucus that has collected throughout the night.
- Children must be discouraged from sucking fingers, using fingers as toothpicks or to clean up and scratch itchy ears. Fingers collect dirt from one surface to the other and can transmit diseases from one part of the body to the other or from one person to the next.

Care of the teeth

Children gain and loose teeth during their early years in school. A child will loose about four teeth per year starting with the first tooth to erupt. Permanent teeth start erupting in six year olds starting with molar teeth. By the age of thirteen, a child should have twenty-eight teeth. As teeth erupt, the shape of the child's jaw and the facial appearances change.

Health care advice

Dental problems in particular tooth decay or dental carries and gum disease may occur at any time without warning.

Children must be advised to maintain a good diet that has low sugary foods. Frequent nutritious snacks, fruit, milk and milk products are good for healthy teeth. A good smile is only possible with clean healthy teeth. Teeth do a lot for an individual, like munching through the three meals a day plus the extra snacks in between meals. Teeth deserve frequent attention.

Care of the mouth should start early in life. It is important to take interest in the health of children's teeth. As the temporary teeth fall off and are replaced by the permanent set, it is important to see how the new set of teeth is growing.

Children should be encouraged to brush teeth after meals. Toothpaste and a good toothbrush have an important role in prevention of tooth decay and strengthening of the teeth. Such information is important to the child so that the child grows up observing healthy habits and can pass the information to the parents who can ensure that the child has these items. Where possible, the tooth- brush must be changed at least every three months.

It is important to regularly inspect the children's teeth to identify such problems as unusually *large teeth*, too *wide gaps* in between the teeth, *teeth growing on top of each other* crowding gums. When these problems are noted, parents can be alerted so that they can take children to health personnel for advice.

Children should be advised to brush teeth thoroughly after every meal using a good toothbrush. The *mouth must be rinsed* with a lot of water to wash away the tiny particles of food that would otherwise remain in the mouth causing a nasty smell and causing tooth decay.

It is wise to *invest in the natural set of teeth*. A diet that is rich in *calcium* and *magnesium* like milk and milk products, fruit and green vegetables is advisable to keep teeth strong.

Sweets and cakes, which are children's favourites, can cause tooth decay. Children should be advised to brush teeth thoroughly after eating these to remove the sugar, which attracts germs that cause tooth decay.

Bad habits

- Teeth should not be used as bottle openers or used as a pair of scissors or knife. This chips and cracks the teeth, weakening them.
- Children must be advised against sucking ice cubes. This habit can cause cracks and chips in teeth and weaken them.

Dental check up

Children must visit a dentist or be seen by a health professional twice a year to get their teeth attended to. Local health personnel from the local clinic can help where a dentist is not available. This yearly check enables evaluation and correction of teething such as gaps in teeth and other alignment problems to prevent potential problems and improve dental appearance.

- The visit to the dentist helps to get problems with the mouth and teeth and one's health in general attended to early.
- It is not wise to wait until one has a toothache to visit a dentist. A dentist does a lot more than tooth extraction. Dentists are happy to attend to chipped teeth, a rotten tooth, or gaps in the mouth at any given time.
- A dentist can help clean stained teeth to enhance one's looks with a beautiful smile. It is also possible for health professionals to pick on other diseases in the body just by looking into the mouth.

- Early forms of *cancer* in the mouth can be identified and treatment can be started early before the cancer spreads.

- *Diabetes* can be identified through a dry mouth and a typical smell that one may not be aware of but the health personnel can pick.

- Children with low levels of iron in their blood, resulting in *anaemia*, often have a dry and pale mouth as well as a sore tongue instead of a pink mouth and pink tongue. This can easily be picked through that dental check up.

- *HIV infection* has special features in the mouth like thrush, bleeding gums and sores in the mouth. More complex diseases like diseases of the bones can also be identified.

Q.E.

1) Do any of the children in your school have problems with their teeth? Discuss with your colleagues how you can arrange for all children to get an annual dental check up.

2) Find out how your pupils look after their teeth on a day-to-day basis and advise accordingly.

3) Can all your pupils afford toothbrushes and toothpaste? Discuss with your class and your colleagues how dental care can be improved for everyone in the school.

4) Discuss with your colleagues strategies to improve the general outlook of your students in your school.

Chapter 5

FOOD AND HEALTH

As a child grows, his/her appetite improves and a healthy child wants to eat frequently because his body organs are growing, his bones are lengthening; his muscles are increasing in length and amount. These changes in body structure require a good diet. Besides, a healthy child is a busy child as he is active playing all day and therefore burns a lot of energy. It is important that parents ensure a good choice of food and appropriate preparation of the food so that a child has a balanced diet and three full meals a day for maximum developmental opportunity. A child who has been deprived of these basic nutritional needs may not enjoy as much good health as the one who has had access to good nutrition.

A poor diet in early life affects the general development of the child physically, mentally and emotionally. Children will eat foods that parents encourage them to eat especially if they are given information on why the type of food is good for them. **Example:** A child who is given information that milk makes one strong will always want his glass of milk because children love to be strong and display their strength when they play with their peers. Many children will not eat green vegetables happily, they need to understand why they must eat them. Similarly children can be discouraged to eat junk food. Emphasis on a balanced diet and reinforcement on basic hygiene contributes positively to a healthy development.

Malnutrition

This is when a child has too little to eat that he/she becomes thin and underweight.

Nutrition and Metabolism

- There is need for a balanced diet to meet growth needs.
- A child needs at least 2400calories spread over the three meals with snacks in between.

- It must be noted that television and radio have strong influence on children's eating habits
- Discuss with children what they want to eat, what they must eat and what they will eat. Parents must always impress on intake of foods rich in iron and vitamin C

Obesity

Obesity is caused by dietary factors common among the affluent populations. Obesity is also associated with some genetic factors and hormonal factors affecting the child's metabolism. This is a problem across all cultures.

A child who has too much to eat and becomes overweight is considered to be malnourished. Children may become malnourished especially where parents are not particularly careful about what their children eat. Liberal parents may contribute to obesity of their children.

- The obese child is likely to develop diabetes, kidney diseases, heart diseases and respiratory diseases because of the strain of the body mass on these systems.
- An obese child may find it difficult to participate in sport and games other children engage in.
- It may be necessary to liase with parents and health personnel to assist the child to loose weight and maintain a weight that is recommended for the age.
- Parents may be advised to monitor what child eats, and encourage the child to take a diet that has reduced fatty foods, reduced carbohydrate foods, controlled fizzy and sugary drinks, sweet dishes, cake and biscuits.
- The child should be encouraged to eat lots of fruit and vegetables and engage in as many sporting activities as possible.
- Parents should consult with health personnel to exclude metabolic disease
- Obesity may result in ridiculing by peers causing low self-esteem, isolation and poor performance in school.

- The child may feel lonely as other children may call him names and this may affect his participation in learning.

Undernourishment

Children may become underweight because of genuine lack of food in extreme poverty, in wars, in droughts and unemployment of parents and lack of land to grow crops.

- An undernourished child may find it difficult to concentrate on schoolwork may have a poor memory and therefore may become a slow learner.
- The undernourished child is prone to illness and infections like chest infections, skin diseases and gastro-intestinal diseases, especially because her/his system may lack essential elements that build immunity to infection.
- The schoolteacher may consult with parents and organizations with interest in the welfare of children for food supplements.
- Parents should be advised to liaise with health personnel who are likely to advise parents on healthy eating, encourage frequent meals for the child and exclude underlying health problems like worm infestation and malabsorption problems.
- Both the obese child and the undernourished child are likely to develop health problems.
- If children are empowered with information on the correct food groups and the contents of their diet, they may be able to make choices on some of the healthy foods.

Eating Disorders

While children may not be very particular about the foods they eat and need advice and close monitoring in the early years of life, eating problems and disorders usually manifest themselves in adolescence.

- The teenager may wish to emulate known and famous characters, and may associate loss of weight mistakenly with beauty.

- Teenagers must be advised that poor eating affects the development of the muscular-skeletal system, causes electrolyte imbalance, and lowers one's immunity and resistance to diseases.
- Eating disorders such as **bulimia nervosa** are becoming more and more common among the adolescent.
- Bulimia is extreme starvation that deprives the body of essential nutrients for adequate blood levels, and mineral salts especially calcium.
- Bone development is affected resulting in contracted and brittle pelvic bones.
- Children and young adults must be encouraged to eat nutritious food and provided with guidance on which foods are good for their health.
- Children must be advised to seek more information on advertised foods on television and other forms of media, as some of them may not necessarily be the best, and some could be the source of obesity.
- Information on healthy eating and especially ability to constitute a balanced diet from available foods is important as part of health promotion.

Healthy Eating

An individual is as healthy as he eats. One needs to eat healthy throughout life to keep all body systems healthy. Eating well is more important in the early years of life to enable healthy development of the individual and ability to achieve full potential in life.

Keeping healthy involves choosing the right foods always. Children must be encouraged to eat three meals in a day and bring a healthy snack to eat at school. In order to keep healthy, the body needs daily portions of the following:

Protein

The body needs protein to build new tissues like muscle and bones as the child grows and to repair damaged and old tissues. Protein also helps to prevent diseases. Protein forms part of all the different fluids in the body, like blood, tears, and even the mucus from the noses. Protein keeps the nerves and every part of the body healthy!

Sources of protein

First class protein or animal protein can be acquired from red meat, fish, chicken, egg whites, seasonal edible beetles, worms and grasshoppers, milk and milk products.

Second class protein or vegetable protein is found in fresh fruit and vegetables, peas, beans, lentils, nuts and peanut butter.

Vitamins

Vitamins make the body able to stand against infection and fight disease. They promote a healthy and smooth skin, strong gums and teeth. Vitamins make the nerves work smoothly and prevent nervousness. Vitamins promote fast wound healing. They promote normal growth in children. They are good for eyesight.

Sources of vitamins

Vitamins are found in fresh foods, fresh farm produce, and fruits. Hard core fruit e.g. apples and pears also help clean teeth and prevent tooth decay. Vegetables, (green and yellow), potatoes, oily fish, milk and milk products are all sources of vitamins. Vitamins are not stored in the body therefore a daily intake is necessary. Vitamins are lost to some extent in cooking and if fruit is cut and left standing for too long.

N.B. When cooking vegetables, it is best to steam them, stir-fry them or boil for a few minutes to prevent destroying the vitamins. If vegetables are boiled thoroughly until they are brown, all vitamins are destroyed by heat.

Fibre

Fibre is the rough strands and threads as well as the husks found in some foods. Fibre prevents constipation and bowel disease e.g. spastic colon and other large bowel problems. Fibre enables the bowels to move frequently and prevents hard stools or constipation. Fibre reduces cholesterol in blood, a substance that causes heart disease.

Sources of fibre

Fibre is found in whole meal foods e.g. whole meal bread, in straight- run maize meal, and whole meal flour. Fibre is available in large amounts in vegetables and hard-core fruit e.g. apples, pears and in fleshy but thready fruit like oranges and mangoes. The tangy sweet sour taste of some fruits e.g. apples; oranges stimulate appetite and also stimulate bowel movement, preventing constipation.

Fluids

The body is made up of 80% water. One must keep on drinking fluids for one's body to stay healthy.

Why does the body need fluids?

The body needs fluids **to make blood** and keep blood flowing to all pats of the body. Blood is life. It carries oxygen (air), food, protection to all parts of the body especially the parts that keep us alive (vital organs) which are the heart, the lungs, the brain, kidneys and the liver. Poor circulation to any part of the body causes death of tissues.

The body needs fluids **to digest food** and for normal bowel movements. Fluids prevent constipation (hard faeces)

The respiratory system (nose, throat and lungs) needs the mucus substance **that traps germs and dust** preventing coughs and lung infection.

Fluids **wash away dirt** and poisons from the body. The kidneys must have enough fluids to get rid of poisons from the body. Without enough fluid one can have disease of the kidneys and bladder (urinary tract infection) and one can have kidney and bladder stones.

The body needs fluids for **other body fluids** such as tears, saliva, and genital fluids.

The internal body parts need water to prevent them from drying up and to continue working normally.

Fluids **cool the body** and prevent high body temperature. Fluids lower body temperature in fevers.

Fluid Loss

The body looses fluid through sweat in high temperatures. It is important to dress lightly in hot weather.

Fluid is lost through bowel movements, urine, vomiting, bleeding, yawning, talking, and singing. The fluids lost in these activities must be replaced to keep healthy.

Without adequate amounts of fluids the body tissues begin to shrivel and dry. Germs attack us especially when our bodies are dry.

Body fluid needs

Adults need **at least two litres of fluid** per day. The body needs more fluid if one is active, sweating, sick and when the weather is hot.

Fluids and children

Children quickly loose fluids and can easily have high temperatures.

Children need plenty of fluids to prevent drying up and showing signs of ill health (dry skin that can be picked between fingers, dry furry tongue, hot body and restlessness, little dark smelly urine).

A child loosing fluid through diarrhea and vomiting must have the fluids replaced.

Children should drink fluids after every meal and when it is hot.

Encourage children to carry water when travelling. **Children must have bottles of water and other nourishing fluids** (fruit juice) when going to school or for games.

Fluids to avoid

Sugary drinks (fizzy drinks like coke and fanta contain high levels of sugar which are likely to cause obesity in children.)

Minerals

Minerals are an important part of the diet. Some of the important minerals are:

Calcium

Calcium is important for building and maintaining healthy bones, teeth, muscles and nerves. In the young, calcium is important to build strong bones and teeth. It is important for healthy function of muscles and nerves. Calcium is needed everyday to maintain the healthy teeth and bones and to prevent holes in the teeth. It is essential for repair of bones after accidents. In the senior members of society, calcium prevents bone thinning and weakening and prevents those bone aches, bone chipping, and fractures. Calcium is found in milk and milk products like yoghurt and cheese. A glass of milk everyday keeps the doctor away! Calcium is found in cereals, in fruits such as bananas, and in vegetables.

Iron

Iron is important for healthy blood. When your blood is healthy, it can prevent attacks from diseases and can fight diseases. Everyone needs iron in his or her blood. Women especially and girls after puberty need a lot of iron to replace blood lost monthly in menses.

Iron can be found in breakfast cereals including the maize-meal porridge and peanut butter, which is full of iron, energy, vitamins and fibre, dried fruit, dried vegetables dried fish, red meat, fruit, (fresh or dried), like apples, pears, and fruit juices, unpolished rice. Iron is also present in milk and other milk products like yoghurt, cheese, sour milk, and ice cream.

Iron is found in large amounts in green leafy vegetables like spinach, cabbage, lettuce and the various types of rape, also, green beans, broccoli, brussel sprouts, beetroot, mushrooms. Ideally it is wise to include something green as part of each meal. Green vegetables add bulk to the diet, help bowels to move and prevent cancer of the bowel.

Starch/Carbohydrates

Starch is essential for energy. Starch is found in large amounts in maize meal, flour, bread, potatoes, rice, pasta, sugar. Starch can be converted to fats and stored in the body as fat. It is wise to eat starch according to the amount of energy one requires. Example: A person who works in the fields all day, or lifts heavy bags all day will need more starch than a person who sits behind a desk all day. When one eats more starch than the body needs, starch is stored in the body in muscles and excess is stored under the skin of thighs buttocks and abdomen as fat where it can be reached when the body needs it.

Fats

Fats are essential fuel foods that generate warmth especially in the cold months. Fats are found in such foods as fatty meats, fried foods, oils, butter. These foods contain lots of calories and fat. Fats can be converted from excess starches. There is therefore no need to eat lots of fatty foods.

If the various groups of foods as outlined above are included in one's diet everyday, it is possible to prevent under nutrition. Children should have at least three balanced meals a day that is breakfast, lunch and supper. A snack in between meals is advisable as children are active and burn up their energy quickly.

N.B.

- A hungry child may not concentrate in class, may sleep, is lethargic and slow in his work.
- A perpetually hungry child may look thin, have a dry rough skin may have a stunted growth, and is slow in class.

Q.E.

1) Ask your pupils to list the foods they have for breakfast, lunch and supper. Help your pupils analyse each meal so that they know the nutritional content of each meal. Give advice on constituting a balanced meal where possible with available affordable foods.

2) Ask health personnel at the local clinic to help in identifying under nourished children. Arrangements can be made for the parents to meet with health personnel for further discussion on the health of the child and depending on the cause they can be referred to the social welfare, or any such organizations with the welfare of children at heart.

Chapter 6

COMMON AILMENTS IN THE SCHOOL AGE CHILD

Infectious diseases are transmitted from one person to another and have a tendency of affecting several people at one time (epidemics) especially in crowded areas such as schools or communities. Common infectious diseases that affect the school child are discussed in this chapter.

THE COMMON COLD (CORYZA)

This is a viral infection that affects especially the respiratory system. Predisposing factors are not clear as the infection is known to affect all age groups, including the healthy looking.

Symptoms

Illness is abrupt and starts with a scratchy and dry feeling on the throat, itchy ears, followed by sneezing, running nose, headache and general body weakness. There is a rise in body temperature up to 38-39c. A dry cough may be present due to the irritation of the throat, tightness in the chest may occur. Within three days, the symptoms should begin to ease. The nasal secretions thicken, and one begins to feel better.

Complications may follow due to bacterial infection causing blocked sinuses, earache, (eustachitis), tonsillitis, inflammation of the large air tubes leading to the lungs, (bronchitis).

Other serious infections like measles, diphtheria, meningitis and whooping cough may present with similar symptoms as the common cold in the early stages of the illness. If one is not sure of the symptoms, it is best to refer the child to the nearest health facility.

Treatment

There is no specific treatment for the common cold. Bed rest should be encouraged for the child. A mild pain relief can be given for the headache and to relieve the tightness in the chest. Cough syrups can be given for the dry cough. The child must be encouraged to take plenty of fluids to reduce the temperature and flush out the infection. The common cold is not treated with antibiotics. Antibiotics can only be used if the doctor confirms the presence of bacterial infection.

Prevention of Spread of the infection

The common cold is spread by droplet infection which occurs quite easily as one infected child sneezes or coughs and droplets of saliva and mucus fly all over in a class. Children must therefore be encouraged to sneeze into hankies or tissue paper. They must be discouraged from spitting in the open.

When a child is infected, he must be encouraged to stay at home until the fever and other symptoms ease.

MUMPS

This is an infectious **viral infection** of the salivary glands.

Transmission

- Mumps is spread by **droplet infection** and direct contact with the saliva of an infected person.
- Mumps occurs mostly in heavily populated areas and may occur in epidemics in crowded places like schools.
- Mumps affects the age groups of between five and fifteen usually in winter months.
- Occasionally mumps occurs in young adults and may be associated with HIV.
- The **virus enters an individual through the mouth**.
- It is found in the saliva within one to six days after infection and before the glands swell.
- Once the virus is in the body, it can enter into the blood system, the kidneys and the spinal cord.

Symptoms and signs

After two to three weeks of infection,

- The infected child feels chills, headaches, general body weakness, and a mild fever.

- The child feels pain on swallowing fluids. Chewing becomes very difficult.
- There is pain on touching the angle of the jaw.
- There is swelling of the salivary glands extending to the cheeks, below the ear, and sometimes to the neck within two days
- In young men, swelling of the testes may occur.
- In severe cases, convulsions and coma may occur.
- Hearing may be affected.

Complications

Some complications that can occur in other parts of the body are:
- Swelling of the pancreas (pancreatitis)
- Swelling of testes (orchitis)
- Inflammation of the kidney (nephritis)
- Inflamation of the covering of the heart (pericarditis)
- Swelling of the thyroid gland (thyroiditis)(Merck Manual, 2002)

Immunity

The chances of repeat infections are rare since one attack of mumps usually gives one immunity thereafter.

General Care

There is no specific treatment for viral infections. Treatment is according to symptoms.
- The child must remain isolated on bed rest until the temperature and swelling have subsided.
- The child must be given lots of fluids to cool the body and keep the temperature low.
- The child must remain isolated from other children until the temperature and swelling have subsided.
- Mild drugs such as aspirin and panadol can be used to reduce pain and swelling according to the child's age.
- A soft diet reduces the discomfort that can be caused by chewing.

Prevention

- An infected child must be isolated to prevent spreading the disease to other children.
- Children must be taught the basic hygienic practices of covering their mouths when sneezing, coughing, and yawning to prevent saliva from flying across to other children.
- Habits such as spitting everywhere must be strongly discouraged.
- Children can also be groomed to keep their mouths closed except when talking.

TONSILLITIS

This is swelling of the tonsils, the two fleshy lumps of tissue on each side of the throat. Tonsils can only be seen below the back of the mouth when one opens the mouth wide.

Causes

Tonsillitis can be caused by bacteria, especially (streptococci), or virus especially following the common cold. The infection is spread by droplet. Epidemics can occur in schools.

Symptoms and Signs

The affected child complains of a sore throat and pain that extends to the ears. There is difficulty in swallowing; vomiting, and some children may refuse to eat. The child also has headache, general body weakness, a high temperature and a bad breath.

The tonsils look red and swollen. In bacterial infection, there may be a white pussy discharge and a white easily breakable, thin membrane spread over the tonsil.

Management

- The affected child should be encouraged to rest in bed.
- Warm throat gargles using mouthwash, salty water, or aspirin dissolved in water should be encouraged to clean up the throat of any pus and reduce the bad smell from the mouth, as well as relieve pain and swelling.
- A mild pain relief should be given for headache.

- A warm bath or sponging will reduce the temperature.
- Antibiotics are given in bacterial tonsillitis to treat infection, clear the pus and prevent its spread to the lungs and ears.

Tonsillectomy or surgery to remove the tonsils is usually considered where there is repeated infection, or in cases where only a brief relief is achieved after antibiotic treatment.

Complications

Repeated bacterial infection may cause serious complications such as:
- Bacterial endocarditis(inflammation of the inner lining of the heart
- Otitis media (inflammation of the inner ears)
- Pneumonia(inflamed lungs)
- Rheumatoid arthritis (swelling of joints).

Diet

A soft diet such as fortified porridge, mashed potato, mashed pumpkin, puddings, soups, and ice-cream can be given until the throat heals and swelling has subsided. The child should be encouraged to take plenty of fluids. Warm drinks are particularly soothing. Fruits such as bananas, grapes, oranges, and fruit juices are especially good for repair of tissues.

SCABIES

This is skin infection caused by the itch mite or **Sacoptes Scabei.**
The mite is found in the dust.
- When children play, the mite attaches itself onto the soft skin folds of the hands, the buttocks, and groins especially. In about an hour the mite will have burrowed its way into the skin causing itchiness.
- The male and female mate on the skin surface and the fertilized mite lives in the burrow where she lays eggs.
- The eggs hatch in three to four days. In a few days the females burrow into the skin and lay more eggs.

- As the infected individual scratches, the skin is further irritated and an itchy pussy rash may occur. Itching is worse at night when the mite gets out of the burrow.

Transmission

The spread of scabies is through skin contact and is more likely in children who share bedding.

Scabies can also be found in adults.

Treatment

- Scabies can easily be treated using topical medicinal substances applied directly to the skin after a warm bath.
- The topical medicine should be left in place for at least twelve hours without washing. It is best to apply on the whole body taking special care of the skin folds.

Prevention

- Children must be thoroughly washed after play taking special attention to skin folds as well as investigating complaints or observation of itch and scratching seriously.
- It is best for children not to share the same bedding as skin diseases can easily be passed onto another child.

RINGWORM

This is infection of the skin and hair caused by fungi.

Types of ringworm

Tinea corporis, affects the skin and can be found on the face, abdomen, back , legs and arms. It looks like round skin lesions or skin patches with raised boarders. It makes the skin itch and one scratches all the time.

Tinea Pedis, or ring worm of the feet, (Athlete' foot).

- This is particularly common even in adults. Infection starts in between the toes but later spreads to the sole of the foot.

- Infection is most common in warm weather. The affected toes become painful and itchy with large amounts of wet dead skin forming under and in between toes.
- The affected soles become thickened and scaly.

Tinea Capitis or ringworm of the scalp

Tinea Capitis affects mainly children although adults can also be affected.

- The hair is broken.
- The lesions are scaly, bold patches extending all over the scalp.
- Affected area of the scalp looks dry and patchy.

Treatment

- Treatment for all ringworm is with anti-fungal drugs and local ointments.
- It is best to seek advice from health personnel from the local health facilities.

Prevention

Ringworm can easily be passed on from one person to the other through contact.

- Encourage children to wash their hair and oil their scalps after playing with dust, and at least daily. Plated hair should also be washed and oiled.
- Advise children not to exchange hats and combs.
- Where possible sharing bed linen should be discouraged.
- Daily bath Is encouraged before retiring to bed, as children arc active throughout the day.
- After washing, the toes must be wiped dry. Bath towels should not be shared.
- Clothes should not be shared.

PEDICULOSIS

This is infestation by **lice**. Infestation may involve the head (pediculus humanus capitis), the body, (pediculus humanus corporis), or the pubis, (phthirus pubis).

Transmission

- Infestation is common where there is **poor hygiene** or where facilities for clean clothing are unavailable.
- Pediculosis is common in **crowded places**.
- Head louse is spread by **direct contact** with an infected person or through hats and combs.
- There is itching and tickling as the lice crawl on the scalp, the body and or pubis. The affected individual scratches incessantly. Itching can be so severe that it becomes distressing.
- On inspecting the scalp or the pubis, small greyish nits can be seen attached to the scalp and hair, sometimes in large numbers. They are difficult to dislodge.
- In three to fourteen days, nits become lice, which can be seen crawling.
- Body lice are found in seams of clothes. The nits are found stuck in the seams of clothes and look small and shiny. They feed on blood and often make lesions on the abdomen, shoulders, and buttocks.

Pediculosis pubis is transmitted sexually.

- The lice are found on the pubic hair, and the fine hairs on the ano-genital region.
- The lice bite and break the skin to feed on blood making the skin itchy. The lice keep warm all over the body under the clothes
- They lay eggs (nits) in the seams of clothes and in the hair. Nits stick on the clothes and hair as they grow.

To prevent lice infestation

- Wear clean and ironed clothes all the time
- Lice and nits from clothes may stick to the body or clothes
- Do not use a friend's comb, nits stick on the comb and can be passed on to a friend
- If one has lice or nits on their clothes or hair, the hair must be cut short, or shaved off. The scalp must be washed clean
- Clothes must be soaked in hot water, washed with soap and ironed.
- Bedclothes too must be soaked in hot water, washed and ironed.

- Lice and nits from clothes may stick to the body or clothes
- Children must be discouraged from using a friend's comb, nits stick on the comb and can be passed to the next person
- Exchanging clothes should be discouraged.
- If one has lice or nits on their clothes or hair, the hair must be cut short, or shaved off.
- The scalp must be washed clean
- Clothes must be soaked in hot water, washed with soap and ironed.
- Bedclothes too must be soaked in hot water, washed and ironed.

Treatment

The hair is best shaved, the head shampoed,1% gamma benzene hexachloride can be applied daily for two days.

The clothes must be soaked and washed in hot water, and ironed with a hot iron.

Prevention

- Children should not exchange clothing items to include shirts, dresses, and hats.
- Children should not exchange or borrow combs.
- Clothes must always be washed thoroughly and ironed before use.
- Where possible, children must not share bedding.

TUBERCULOSIS

Tuberculosis is a long-term infection caused by the **Mycobacterium Tuberculosis**.

Transmission

Tuberculosis is almost always caught through inhalation. The bacteria are often not trapped by the mucous membrane of the nostrils and the rest of the upper respiratory system and often move down to reach the lungs without being trapped.

Tuberculosis can be confined to the respiratory system or it can be spread to other parts of the body.

Pulmonary Tuberculosis, (lung tuberculosis), is briefly described in this book.

Pulmonary Tuberculosis

- Tuberculosis occurs mostly in crowded, unhygienic places like slums, army barracks, school dormitories, and in low socio-economic communities.
- Tuberculosis is also an opportunistic infection affecting those people already weakened by other diseases like those with long standing pneumonia, severe malnutrition, HIV, to name but a few.
- The bacteria sit at the base of the lung where it destroys lung tissue causing cavities in the lungs.

Symptoms and Signs

The symptoms and signs of tuberculosis **do not appear immediately** and may take a long time to surface.

- The individual feels a general body weakness, low grade fever, loss of appetite and loss of weight.
- Later, one has **a cough**, most troublesome in the morning
- As the disease progresses, the cough becomes marked throughout the day.
- One coughs up **greenish pussy sputum** and as blood vessels are eroded by the cavities, the sputum becomes bloody.
- The blood in sputum may be massive depending on the size of blood vessel affected.
- There is **severe chest** pain especially when breathing. There is **breathlessness**.
- The progress of the disease depends on the individual's resistance and also on early commencement of treatment.

Complications that can occur

- One can have collection of fluid in the chest, **pleural effusion**, a very painful condition that restricts expansion of the lungs as one breathes in.
- One can have **lung collapse** (atelectasis) meaning that one's lung can no longer expand to contain the much needed life-sustaining oxygen.
- Tuberculosis can spread to other parts of the body.
- **Tuberculosis kills**.

Advice on Prevention and Control of Tuberculosis

- All children should be vaccinated with the BCG vaccine against tuberculosis.

- Mild chest infections must be thoroughly treated to prevent general deterioration of health.

- If one child in the school is infected, it is important that his classmates and suspected communities and contacts of infected persons are screened for possible infection.

- Tuberculosis is **HIGHLY INFECTIOUS**. Children are advised not to spit everywhere. If one must spit. It must be in a hanky or tissue which is properly disposed of.

- The school teacher should take special interest in children with loss of weight, persistent cough, and those who may become unduly breathless on minimal effort such as during normal play with other children and during sporting activities. The children should be screened for tuberculosis.

- Infected child **must be isolated** until he/she is no longer infectious. This is after tests of sputum that indicate the absence of the bacterium in the sputum. Take interest in the laboratory results of the infected.

- People should be encouraged to improve their houses by building spacious rooms with large windows to allow air to circulate.

- It is important for communities to improve their general hygiene to prevent the spread of the disease.

- Improvement of nutrition and a balanced diet is essential to prevent opportunistic diseases.

Treatment

Tuberculosis can be treated if it is diagnosed early. The treatment is a long-term treatment but must be adhered to or else the individual can be re-infected and the diseases spread to family members and those closest to the individual such as classmates.

Reference

Merck Manual of Diagnosis and Therapy (2006) 18th Ed.

Chapter 7

WATER BORNE DISEASES

These are diseases caused by a host that requires the presence of water to carry on fuelling disease.

Bilharzia

Bilharzias is caused by a small, flat, leaf-like worm called **Schistosoma Haematobium** when in urine and **Schistosoma Mansoni** when in the bowel. The worm can only be seen by a microscope.

- The bilharzial worm lives partly in man where it enters by burrowing through the skin when one bathes in or wades through stagnant waters.
- The worms travel through blood veins to the liver where they develop and mate. The female finds its way to the veins of the bladder or bowel where she deposits her eggs.
- Eggs may be deposited in the spinal cord causing paralysis. The period between infection and laying eggs is ten to twelve weeks.
- The eggs are passed through urine and faeces. They hatch into small worms called **miracidium**, which quickly find their host, the snail, within eight hours. In four to six weeks the snail gets rid of a worm the **cercariae**.
- An infected snail will continue to shed the cercariae for about a year.
- Cercariae can live for up to 48hours swimming freely in stagnant water looking for a host, a person or an animal.
- An itchy rash may appear where the cercariae has burrowed through a person's skin.

Effects in the affected

- Bilharzias can cause general ill health. Six to eight weeks after infection, a child may have a high temperature, cough and an enlarged swollen liver.
- Dullness and sluggish thinking can be suggestive of bilharzial infection. The child may also have unexplained loss of weight.

- Blood is lost in varying amounts as the cercaria burrows throw body tissues and as the adult worm feeds in the veins of the bladder and bowel.

- Nerves of the bladder and bowel can be affected causing poor control of the bladder and bowel.

- Blood can be seen at the end after passing urine or faeces. This repeated bleeding causes long-term anaemia. The presence of the adult worms can cause local changes in the bowel and bladder.

Control of bilharzia

Snail Control.

- Efforts can be made to clear ponds of snails by stocking the ponds with fish to eat the cercariae and ducks to eat the snails.

- Environmentalists can use chemicals to clear the snails.

Control of bad habits

- Man can be prevented from infecting the snail by careful disposal of faeces and urine in latrines and water closets. Free flowing urine and freely deposited faeces can be swept into water ponds in the rainy season continuing the bilharzial cycle.

- Children should be warned and prevented from wading, swimming, bathing in snail infested stagnant waters.

- Communities should be encouraged and advised to use clean domestic water from taps, deep protected wells and boreholes.

- Drinking water should be boiled and cooled before drinking. Bath water should be boiled before use.

- Parents should be encouraged to ensure that the children have shoes especially in the rainy seasons.

- Makeshift bridges of stone or logs can be put across swamps so that as the children cross these swamps, they are not in contact with the potentially infected water.

Q.E.1) Can your pupils identify a pond close by the school? Go through the stages of bilharzial infection with them and let them discuss the possibility of the pond as a source of bilharzias. Let them suggest ways of making the pond safe and assist them to make the suggestions a reality.

2) How many of your pupils wade through shallow waters on their way to school? Can you help them make a makeshift bridge across the shallow waters by mobilizing either the local community or the class?

3) Do you think any of the children in your class could have bilharzia? Refer the child to the local health centre for tests. If the results are positive, use this case to encourage the local community to do something about the possible source of infection before many pupils are infected.

MALARIA

Malaria is caused by the parasite **plasmodium falciparum** carried by the female anopheles mosquito.

- The anopheles mosquito lays its eggs in sun warmed slow moving or stagnant water, and in any containers that can hold water.

- The adult mosquito lives in tall grass, in dark corners of the buildings and anywhere it can find shelter.

- The plasmodium multiplies in the mosquito gut. The oocytes or the little worms so formed develop to become sporozites which move to the salivary glands of the mosquito.

- As the infected mosquito feeds on human and animal blood, the sporozites are released into the blood of the human or animal.

- Within thirty minutes after being introduced in the blood, the sporozites can be found in the liver, the spleen and the bone marrow where they grow and mature.

- The mature sporocytes release trophozoites, which invade red blood cells and develop to become schizoints.

- When mature, schizoints release numerous merozoites causing the destruction of the red cell. As more and more red cells are attacked the typical malaria picture of chills, fever and sweating occurs.

- Some of the merozoites develop into gametocytes, which are picked by the mosquito as it drinks blood from the infected person. The cycle starts again and takes about three weeks to be complete, while the mosquito can live for a further three weeks.

- The result of the infection is a reduction in red blood cells causing anaemia. The damaged red cells stick together causing clots, cerebral malaria, liver failure, kidney failure, and passing bloody urine **(black water fever).**

- Malaria kills due to the high fever, the destruction of red cells and the changes occurring in the vital organs of the body.

- Should you suspect that a child has malaria, send the child to the clinic immediately for treatment. The course of the treatment must be finished for the treatment to be effective.

- Advise the child to drink a lot of fluids to cool the body and wash out as much wastes as possible from the body systems.

Protection against Malaria

Travel

- Before one visits mosquito-infested areas, one must take protection in the form of tablets that can be taken at least one week before the visit. These can be found in chemists and   local clinics.

- After visiting a malarial area one should go for a blood test and seek advice from the local health centre.

Clear environment

- Children can be advised to clear all the rubbish around the home and at the school.

- Papers and plastics must be burnt or collected into bags to be handed to companies that recycle paper .

- Empty tins must be broken so that they cannot hold water, broken cups and bottles that hold water must be collected and disposed of safely or buried in the ground.

- Grass around homes should be kept short so that it does not attract mosquitoes.

Mosquito repellents

- Insecticides in the form of aerosols or coils can be used in the homes to kill adult mosquitoes. Insecticides should be kept away from the reach of children.
- Spraying should be done at least two hours before people go to sleep to prevent chemical inhalation and respiratory failure. Where public health spray teams treat the whole environment, it is best for houses to be sprayed in the morning.
- The sprayed houses must be thoroughly cleaned to prevent respiratory accidents, as the chemical concentrations are higher than those found in commercial aerosol cans.
- Houses sprayed must be kept open for at least six to eight hours before they can be used.
- The skin can be oiled and creamed with mosquito repellents in the evenings.

Clothing

After dark, people should wear long sleeved clothes and long dresses/trousers to protect themselves from mosquito bites.

Mosquito Nets

- Treated mosquito nets that cover up the whole length of bed at night must be used by both children and adults.

Paint choice

- White paint or light coloured paint in buildings limits the presence of mosquitoes because mosquitoes favour dark surfaces where they can blend with the walls and are not easily identified.

Fans

- A fan prevents mosquitoes from sitting on a surface and where these are affordable, they should be left on all night.

Attention to sources of water

- Stagnant waters can be covered with a film of paraffin or a recommended insecticide to destroy the eggs of the mosquito.
- Small ponds of water must be drained and pits that hold water filled with soil.

Q.E.

1) After discussing malaria with pupils, the teacher can ask pupils to go round the school and identify anything they may associate with mosquito breeding and arrange for action to be taken to minimize breeding of mosquitoes such as collection of empty bottles and tins, cutting grass, filling up pits and holes that hold water with sand. Ensure that pupils take active participation and encourage them to go and repeat the activity at their homes.

2) Ask the pupils to share the activities they were involved in at home to prevent mosquito breeding.

Reference

1. Merck Manual of Diagnosis and Therapy (2006) 18th Ed. Merck

Chapter 8

DISEASES CAUSED BY CONTAMINATED FOOD

Diarrhoeal diseases

Diarrhoea is an increase in fluidity, volume and frequency of bowel movements. Different diseases are identifiable by the amounts of faecal material passed at any given moment, its consistency, the presence of pus or blood, mucus and fatty material.

Causes of diarrhoea

Causes of diarrhoea in children are many.

- Children have a tendency to eat raw fruit, chew dirty pencils, pick things from the ground and eat food without washing hands. These habits and many more can cause ingestion of varied amounts of germs that upset the digestive system.
- Diarrhoea can be caused by poisons (toxins) of ingested bacteria such as in cholera, shigellosis, typhoid, food poisoning, (botulism), and mal-absorption.

The effect of diarrhoea on the body

The small and large bowel, normally absorb water from the bowel into the blood vessels and the body.

- In all diarrhoeas, the toxins or poisons from the micro-organisms in the bowel, cause fluid to be absorbed from the body into the bowel only to be eliminated from the body.
- The withdrawal of fluid from body tissues into the bowel for excretion results in the loss of salts (electrolytes) such as sodium, potassium, organic anions, and chlorides from body tissues resulting in severe loss of fluid and dehydration, circulatory failure and collapse.

Signs of dehydration are :

- A person that has had several diarrhoeal motions has a hot, dry and wrinkled skin that can be "picked" on pinching, especially on the abdomen, the arms and thighs.
- A person with severe diarrhoea has shortness of breath causing sighing or gasping for air.
- The person has severe body weakness.
- The person's tongue becomes dry and furred and the individual may complain of severe thirst.

Treatment

Diarrhoea is only a symptom of an underlying disorder. The cause of the problem has to be investigated.

- The affected individual must be quickly referred to a health facility before complications like severe dehydration and collapse occur.
- The lost fluids must be replaced. The individual must be given plenty of oral fluids to replace lost fluid. Salt and sugar solution must be given in large amounts to replace lost electrolytes.
- If the individual is able to eat, food they can be offered easily absorbable foods that contains no fat.

Prevention of spread of disease

- The faecal matter of the infected person must be properly disposed of in a toilet.
- Gloves must be used to prevent contaminating hands.
- Hands must be thoroughly washed after handling the sick or faecal matter.

Prevention of diarrhoeal diseases and their spread in schools:

- All pupils must be encouraged to wash their hands thoroughly after toilet use.
- Pupils must be advised on the use of protected and boiled water, well-cooked food, and safe storage of cooked food to prevent contamination and food poisoning.

Simple hygiene measures must be emphasized.

- Washing hands before handling food
- Washing hands after use of toilet
- Washing hands after shaking hands with many people such as at large community gatherings,
- Washing food thoroughly before cooking,
- Covering food to protect it from flies and dust.

CHOLERA

Cholera is an acute infection of the bowel caused by an organism called **Vibrio cholerae**.

Transmission

Cholera is spread by **ingestion of food and water contaminated by faeces** of an infected person. Cholera affects all age groups exposed to contaminated water or food.

- It takes one to three days after the ingestion of contaminated food for the signs and symptoms to appear.
- As soon as it enters the bowel, vibrio cholerae **produces a poison** that causes large amounts of fluids to be drawn from body tissues and poured into the bowel.
- The accumulation of fluid in the bowel results in a **sudden onset of painless watery diarrhoea and vomiting.**
- The affected individual becomes severely dehydrated, thirsty, and suffers from muscle cramps.
- The individual becomes very weak.
- The skin becomes dry and wrinkled.
- The blood becomes diminished and concentrated.
- The individual passes very little and concentrated urine or no urine at all.
- If untreated, the individual lapses into a coma, has renal failure and heart failure and may die within hours of onset of symptoms.

Treatment

Cholera can be overcome by prompt correction of fluid loss.

- Large amounts of salt and sugar solution should be given by mouth. The individual should be transferred to hospital or health facility quickly where the appropriate fluid replacement treatment and antibiotics will be given.

Prevention

- Faeces should be properly disposed of in the toilets built on lower ground from water sources and at least a hundred metres apart.
- In rural areas, communities should be encouraged to build toilets and use them.
- Hands must be washed after use of toilet, after shaking hands and before handling food.
- Hands must be thoroughly washed pouring water onto the hands and not using a dish or taking turns to wash hands from a dish of water.
- Communities must be encouraged to have clean sources of water such as deep protected wells, boreholes or piped water for their domestic water.
- The source of drinking water should be situated on high ground in the opposite direction from refuse disposal pits and toilets.
- Where the source of water is open, drinking water must be boiled.
- Vegetables must be thoroughly washed before use
- Cholera vaccine should be given in areas where cholera outbreaks are likely to occur

Q.E.

1) Find out what practices of human waste disposal your pupils have at their homes and advise accordingly.

2) Are there facilities in the school for pupils to wash their hands regularly? If not, discuss this with fellow teacher colleagues and the catchments community for the school and seek a way forward.

TYPHOID

Typhoid fever is infection of the bowel by **Salmonella typhi** through **ingestion of contaminated water and food.**

Transmission

- The source of infection is the **faeces of carriers** or **faeces and urine of infected person**.
- Infection can be through contaminated water, vegetables, milk and any other food in communities with poor sanitation,.
- Infection can be through food handlers in the food industry.

Changes in the body of the infected person

- After the salmonella organism gets to the small and large bowel, it burrows into the tissue of the bowel causing ulceration and haemorrhage by the third week of infection.
- Perforation of the bowel may occur resulting in bleeding and spilling of the bowel contents onto the rest of the abdominal contents. This causes severe weakening of the individual and collapse of the individual.

Symptoms and Signs

It takes 3 to 25 days for symptoms and signs to appear depending on the number of organisms ingested.

- The individual feels chills, general body weakness, headache, and loss of appetite, backache, and constipation and may bleed from the nose.
- There is abdominal pain and tenderness.
- The temperature rises daily for seven to ten days then falls gradually.
- A rash appears on the chest and abdomen (the rose spots) with a new rash appearing every three days.
- In the late second week, a thin, greenish, offensive, typical (pea soup) diarrhoea occurs. The individual becomes confused and delirious, and falls into a coma.

Treatment

Typhoid kills if untreated.

- Typhoid can be successfully treated with antibiotics.
- Lost fluid and salts will need to be replaced.
- Recovery is very slow and can take up to three months.

Care of the infected

- The infected person should be isolated and kept on bed rest for a long time.
- If constipated give lots of fluids. Do not give laxatives.
- Wash hands thoroughly after handling the individual or the human waste.
- The individual can only be considered safe if laboratory results confirm his faeces negative of the disease.

Diet

A highly nutritious fluid diet (soups and fruit juices), and soft semi-solid diet (purees and mashed food) should be given.

Prevention

- Communities must be encouraged to observe high standards of hygiene.
- Rural communities must be advised on sighting of toilets.
- Communities must be encouraged to secure a safe and secure source of domestic water such as boreholes, deep protected wells and piped/tap water.
- Hands must be washed after use of toilet, before handling food, after hand shaking with a lot of people.
- Drinking water must be boiled or buy bottled water if not sure of the water source.
- Workers in the food industry must be screened for the bacillus at least every six months.
- Careful choice of restaurants should be made when eating out.
- Raw vegetables (for salads) must be thoroughly washed before use. During epidemics, it may be wise to avoid salads completely.

- Take any cases of diarrhoea seriously and refer them to the local health facility urgently.
- Take interest in the laboratory results of a child who has had diarrhoea so as to be able to advise accordingly.

N.B. Typhoid is highly infectious and a danger to lives.

ANTHRAX

Anthrax is a disease common in animals especially those that graze, like cattle, goats, sheep and horses. Anhrax is caused by an organism called **Bacillus Anthracis**. This is a very resilient micro-organism that is difficult to destroy.

- The microorganism forms a shell and stays in the soil for many years.
- Animals get infected through grazing and if the shell sticks onto the fur as the animal lies down in the pastures.
- Inside the animal the shell breaks open due to the warmth of the body heat. The organism becomes live and active and starts growing.
- As the bacillus grows in the animal it produces a poison that affects the animal.
- Anthrax is common in those animals that are not regularly vaccinated and are not dipped. It may therefore appear in the dry months of the year and immediately after, where animals are left to roam without veterinary attention and dipping.

Transmission to people

- Anthrax is transmitted to people through contact with infected animals or animal products.
- People working with animals like herdsmen, veterinary staff, abattoirs staff and people working with hides are more likely to contract anthrax.

The ordinary person gets anthrax in three ways.

- The most common way is eating **infected meat**, boiled or roasted.
- Eating meat from an animal that has been killed because it was unwell
- Eating meat from animals that have died from an unknown cause.

The anthrax bacillus becomes active as soon as it is inside the individual and *produces a poison*, which weakens the heart muscle. The poison causes **swelling of internal organs.**

The person has

- nausea,
- vomiting
- a very high temperature
- severe body weakness.
- *skin anthrax (cutaneous anthrax)* occurs in most of the people who are infected. A small pimple forms, which soon becomes dark in the centre while its margins are red and swollen. It later oozes a watery bloody fluid. The poison spreads in the body causing swelling of the internal organs.

The pulmonary or inhalation or lung anthrax is inhaled as one breathes.

- The organism multiplies quickly in the chest where there is abundant blood and oxygen.

Pulmonary Anthrax causes:

- severe swelling of lungs,
- collection of fluid in the chest,
- severe chest pain,
- coughing up blood
- difficulty in breathing
- high fever
- Loss of consciousness.

Treatment

Anthrax can be treated with antibiotics if health care is sought early.

Without treatment, **an infected person may die within three to seven days.**

Prevention

- Anthrax can be prevented through vaccination of animals.
- Veterinary workers, abattoir workers, herdsmen, butchers, game rangers and tannery workers are at risk of contracting anthrax and should be vaccinated annually.

- Animals that look unwell **should not be killed for meat**.
- Animals that have died on **their own should not be skinned or eaten** but should be put in a deep pit and burnt.

Reference

1. Merck Manual of Diagnosis and Therapy (2006) 18th Ed. Merck

Chapter 9

CONVULSIONS

Convulsions are characterised by severe shaking of the whole body with or without temporary loss of consciousness.

Causes of Convulsions:

- High temperature like in malaria,
- Lack of adequate amounts of oxygen to the brain especially after strenuous exercise
- Low blood glucose
- food poisoning
- Renal failure .
- Previous injury to the head
- Brain abscess and brain tumor
- **Hysteria.**Some children may mimic convulsions to gain sympathy especially when they are unwilling to take part in activities or as a way of getting attention. The teacher must be able to separate real health problems from hysteria. This chapter will discuss in detail epilepsy.

EPILEPSY

This is commonly referred to as fits.

Epilepsy is a health problem of the brain that affects people of all ages, all races and walks of life.

Epilepsy may be provoked but could also be spontaneous.

There are many forms of this problem differing from one individual to the next.

Epilepsy arises from chemical imbalance in the brain causing sudden brief change in the function of the brain cells.

Depending on which part of the brain is affected, where the chemical imbalance spreads to and the extent of the brain area affected, the affected person will react accordingly.

Causes of Epilepsy

- Epilepsy may or may not have a known cause.

- It can be genetic originating from structural disorders of the brain.
- It can be caused by abnormal nerve development
- It can be due to lack of oxygen to the baby while it grew in the mother's womb or lack of oxygen to the brain after delivery (anoxia).
- Convulsions or fits that occur before a child is two years old could be because of injury at birth, problems in growth affecting the brain, diseases affecting the brain or high body temperatures.
- Fits that occur after the age of two years may not have a known cause or may follow injury and brain tumours (abnormal growths).
- Infection that causes high temperatures such as meningitis may cause convulsions.
- Diseases affecting one area of the brain and nerves like meningitis (swelling of the covering of the brain), tetanus, syphilis, rabies, malaria may cause fits at any age.
- Injury that leaves a tiny scar in the brain such as depressed fracture of the scull in bad falls prevents the smooth function of the brain.
- Epilepsy can be caused by a brain tumour, brain abscess.
- Epilepsy can be caused by conditions such as hypoglycaemia (low blood glucose), hypocalcaemia (low blood calcium), hyponatremia (low blood sodium).
- Epilepsy can also be caused by poisons such as poisonous gases, smoke, illicit drugs, and alcohol.
- In mature people, fits can be caused by the above as well as high blood pressure leading to stroke.
- Epilepsy can be caused by degeneration of nerves such as dementia, Alzheimer's disease.

The fits may only come when the cause is still present. After the condition is treated, in most of these situations the fits will stop. But if there is a permanent scar on the brain, the fits may come repeatedly.

N.B. It must be noted that people with hysteria, especially teenagers and some young adults, may act as if they have fits to get attention and sympathy. The difference between an epileptic fit and a non epileptic attack is as follows:

Features seizure	Epileptic seizure	Non-epileptic seizure
Onset	Sudden	May be gradual
Pelvic thrusting	Rare	Common
Thrashing movements	Rare	Common
Rolling movements	Rare	Common
Cyanosis (blue/grey skin colour due to lack of oxygen)	Common	Unusual
Tongue biting	Common	Less common
Duration	Seconds/minutes	Often many minutes
Gaze aversion	Rare	Common
Resistance to passive limb movements	Unusual	Common
Prevention of leg falling onto face	Unusual	Common
Drowsiness after fit	Usual	Often absent
Blinking movements	Unusual	Present

(Kodabuckus,2010)

Triggers of Fits

- Missing tablets lowers the level of the treatment drug in the body
- Infections and illness raise temperatures and interfere with the usual epileptic drugs
- Photosensitivity e.g. flickering disco lights, sunshine shimmering on water, computers, television, patterns on paper or clothes are irritants to the brain
- Menstruation causes changes in fluid levels in the body and brain causing tension in the brain which triggers convulsions
- Alcohol, stress, boredom, hyperthermia, lack of sleep, missed meals all alter the mood, electrolyte levels in the body triggering fits.
- Diet: High levels of caffeine, tea, cola drinks, aspartate in fizzy drinks are brain stimulants that cause unnecessary excitement in the brain that can trigger fits.

Some known facts about fits

- Fits can be **generalised**, that is the whole body is affected, or they can affect just one limb (**focal** fits).
- It may be possible to tell that a person with fits is about to have an attack as many show warning signs which are:
- Cry (aura)
- Altered consciousness
- Doing unusual, uncontrolled, unplanned behaviours (Automatisms).

Warning Signs Before A Fit

Automatisms are uncontrolled, unplanned behaviours before a fit.

- Alimentary behaviours: Chewing, lip smacking, swallowing,
- Mimicry behaviours: Laughter, fear, anger, excitement
- Gestures: Fiddling with hands, tapping, rubbing, tidying, undressing, genitally directed movements
- Ambulatory movements: walking, circling, running
- Violent behaviour. Any behaviours that the person displays when not restrained is not premeditated.
- Some just **stare blankly** into space as if they are in a trance.
- Some see **flashes of light** and images (hallucinations).
- Some get specific **smells**.
- Deviation of head and eye to one side
- Adoption of a raised flexed arm
- Speech arrest or muttering
- A **loud cry**, **falling** and **loss of consciousness** follow this.

The Fit

- The body muscles become stiff followed by uncontrollable jerking of all muscles including the trunk, neck and head.
- Eyes open widely as the eyeballs are upturned
- The mouth froths, the tongue may be bitten.
- The bladder and bowel may open.
- A deep sleep usually follows.
- On waking up, the individual is confused and does not remember what happened. This stage may be dangerous as the person may wonder about

and injure himself or others while in the state of confusion (**stage of automatism**).

This type of fit may last two minutes to fife minutes.

Some fits may come frequently with one fit following another without the individual gaining consciousness (**status epilepticus***).

Managing a person with a fit

- Seizures can be frightening to onlookers. The individual having seizures is not in pain and will have little or no recollection of what is going on or what happened. If you happen to be close by when one has a fit, or if you live with someone who suffers from fits:

- Remember that **the seizure cannot be stopped** so it is important to let it take place.

- Always be on the alert especially to **pick the signs of a coming fit**. Remove the individual from any objects that may cause him injury. If possible sit him on the floor/ground away from furniture items or other objects.

- When the fits start **do not hold the person** or restrain him but stay close by and observe the type of fit .

- **Loosen tight clothing**

- Remove spectacles

- Stop people from crowding

- **Do Not** **put something in the mouth** to prevent injury this may instead cause the person injury.

- **Do not attempt to restrain movements**

- **Do not give anything to drink until fully awake.**

- **Do not move the person unless the person is in immediate danger** (British National Society for Epilepsy, 1991)

- After the powerful muscular jerking, lie the individual on his side making sure that the chin is pulled forward to prevent the tongue from falling back and blocking free breathing.

- Leave the individual to rest.

- Wipe the saliva away and check the airways

- Protect the person by providing privacy

- Reassure the person until fully conscious.

- When the person wakes up, observe his actions remembering that he may be confused at this stage and may harm himself or others. Talk to him gently, do not frighten him.

- Attend to his injuries if any especially the tongue. Ask him to rinse his mouth clean.

- Ensure that he is on treatment and that he has taken the treatment. If he has not had a fit before, he must be taken to the nearest health facility or doctor for investigations.

N.B An individual who is having one fit after another must be taken to the hospital immediately. This is a dangerous type of fit which may result in loss of life!

Important Points

- Epilepsy cannot be spread from one person to the other. It is therefore safe to touch the individual and to clean him up.

- Evil spirits do not cause epilepsy; so do not be afraid to assist the epileptic. There is no need to engage voodoos and rituals for an epileptic. The doctors can competently manage this condition.

Advice to epileptics

- Medication must be taken everyday according to doctor's orders. The child must carry the medication with them when travelling on school trips and the teacher must be aware of how the medication should be taken. It is possible to live a healthy normal life free of fits as long as they take their medication.

- Parents of children with epilepsy should never agree to be persuaded to stop taking their medication by anyone, a herbalist, a religious prophet or a relative. Medication is the child's life!

- Children suffering from epilepsy should be advised to keep the doctor's appointment whatever happens. It is important that their medication is reviewed regularly and that their health is monitored closely.

- Children suffering from epilepsy are advised to wear a Medic Alert, a small bracelet that tells what one is suffering from. It can be worn around the neck like a necklace or around the wrist like a bracelet. This can serve a life as one can quickly get help.

- The school staff must know about such health problems so that the pupils are not exposed to danger, like swimming pools. By watching the tiny waves in pools of water epileptics may be irritated enough to go into a fit.

- The doctor or clinic can give more information about associations or clubs where parents of children with epilepsy meet with others with similar problems and share ideas. There are many epileptics out there who live happy lives without fits by adhering to their medication and advice.

Lifestyle implications

It is important to distinguish between restrictive and non-restrictive measures based on risk assessment depending on the type of fit an individual has and its triggers to make decisions about lifestyle.

Advice:

Bedroom

A child with epilepsy uses a low bed and not a bunk bed.

There should be basic furniture in the room.

Bathroom

The child should preferably use shower and avoid a tub.

Kitchen

The child is best supervised in the kitchen. An electric stove may be safer than gas.

Travel

It is safer for the child to driven or to use public transport than a bicycle.

In cold months it is safer to use gas heaters or electric heaters than an open fire.

Sports and leisure

Sports which keep the child safe like ball games, sprints would be safe for the child as compared to swimming and jumps.

There is also need for advice when one decides to use contraceptives and when one wants to start a family.

Long term monitoring of Epilepsy

- It is important that one has a seizure diary that describes the frequency of seizures, the duration and pattern of the seizures
- An identification bracelet is important in case one is found unconscious.
- Training of the next of kin on management of a seizure is important.

Reference

2. Kodabuckus,W.(2002) Epilepsy Care. South Birmingham NHS Primary Care Trust.
3. Merck Manual of Diagnosis and Therapy (2006) 18th Ed. Merck

Chapter 10

SEXUAL DEVELOPMENT

The school age child enters school knowing fully well what his/her sex is and may have a strong identification with the parent of the same sex. The child then learns the concepts of behaviours expected of her sex role. The child further develops a curiosity and desire to learn about the biologic aspects of sexual function. It is not uncommon for children of the same sex to explore each other's sexual organs. This is not necessarily homosexual behaviour but more of curiosity.

Children may not be sure whom to ask about the sexual questions they may have and may pass misinformation to their peers. Parents too maybe uncomfortable to give information or may not have the correct information.

The teacher with the help of health personnel has a role in giving sexual health education to the growing child. Health personnel can fill up the gaps and correct misconceptions.

Sexual Health information

Between the ages of six to eleven years most children enjoy reading and writing, counting, drawing and coloring. During this stage, the child draws figures that represent women; mother, sisters and tries to show the difference between the women figures and men; dad and brother. The child can gradually learn how the girl or boy gradually grows, personal development and the subsequent developmental stage, puberty. Age specific books in health can be made available to the child while special attention is paid to explaining and answering questions honestly. The child is also keen to learn tasks appropriate for age and gender.

Body Concept

The 8-11 age group begins to have a body concept. They are fascinated sometimes surprised and worried about changes taking place on their bodies. Children are curious to know about their body parts and the relationship of body organs. Changes and differences in the body often raise a lot of curiosity and questions. Children may also be frightened or embarrassed by body changes. Some changes like obesity, development of breasts, a few hairs in the armpits and pubic area, may bring about ridicule from other children causing embarrassment, loss of friends and withdrawal in the affected child. Parents and teachers can play a major role in helping children learn developmental self- care skills from an early age responding to questions with correct information. Special group education programmes can be arranged to equip the school age child with information and respond to questions the children may have.

Genital mutilation

This is a practice in some countries in which sections of the external female genitalia are excised as a traditional practice.

- The procedure is carried out by elderly women of the community under no form of pain relief to the young girls and subjecting the young girls to excruciating pain, loss of blood and exposure to infection.

- There is no known advantage of this practice to the young girl. This practice is known to cause ugly scars that cause complications in later life especially during child birth.

- Many activists are now lobbying for the abolition of this practice and discouraging the practice through education of the elderly members of society as well as empowering the young girls to stand for their rights and resist the call to be circumcised.

- School teachers should add their voices to that of lobbyists because this practice exposes innocent children without any decision making powers to unnecessary pain and man- made mutilation that will later on affect the girls' sexual life.

- This practice makes child bearing uncomfortable resulting in further injury and difficult child delivery. The pain that the little girls are subjected to is unnecessary. Some children loose lives because of severe bleeding and infection.

There is no reason why any person must remove healthy natural structures of the genital area of little innocent girls.

Sexual Abuse

This is any indecent contact with a child, a person without their consent.
Sexual abuse may be

- Caressing, fondling or grabbing breasts, patting the buttocks, or touching, of any part of the child's body in an indecent way.

- Touching or contact with a child's genital organs

- Penetration of a child's organs and forcibly eliciting sexual intercourse.

- Sexual abuse is usually perpetrated by trusted members of family, and other members of society entrusted with the care of children in schools, children's homes and refugee camps as well as by social deviants and perverts. Abusers are indiscriminate and can abuse both boys and girls.

- Sexual abuse is a serious health problem which has to be reported to police as soon as it is known.
- Sexual abuse is in many forms some of which are briefly described below.

Incest

Incestuous relationships or sexual relationship between related people or close family members are sexual abuse.

- This behaviour may occur in broken homes where a parent replaces the lost partner with one of the children for sexual satisfaction
- Guardians entrusted with the welfare of a minor child end up molesting the child.
- Some misguided family members believe incestuous relationships bring luck in business, in misfortune, and in healing illness.
- Sexual abuse robs the young person of her innocence, confuses the young person who becomes emotionally unstable and looses trust and confidence in members of society and family.
- Young children may be exposed to sexually transmitted diseases including the deadly HIV/AIDS through the sexual abuse.

The school teacher must openly discuss this evil practice that confuses children and destroys their future. The school teacher must encourage children to divulge such practices and be able to identify abused children. These practices must be reported to police, social services and human rights organizations.

Rape

Rape is forced sexual act without the consent of the other partner.

- Rape is an offence and punishable by law.
- Most rape victims show mental trauma.
- The child is often frightened to give an account of the events of the rape.
- The child may be withdrawn or may pretend to be unconcerned.
- Children have to trust the individual asking them about the incident to talk about it.

- They have to be in a relaxed environment without pressure or being hurried.
- Rape victims are scared to be interviewed by a male teacher or to confide in a male health worker as this may bring back memories of the rape.

Children will talk in the presence of an empathetic, non- threatening, non- judgmental female member of staff who can report this crime to police.

Psychological Effect of Sexual Abuse

- Most abusers will use persuasion and may give the child sweets and any such things to spoil the child and keep the child quiet.
- The child may be made to believe that the abuser is a special friend and that what they do is their secret, which should never be known by other people.
- On the other hand a close member of the family may use threats, intimidation, and dangerous weapons, such as a gun or a knife and extreme violence to intimidate the child to keep quiet.
- Abusers tend to repeat the abusive act over and over. A child can be abused for years without divulging the abuse.
- Sometimes the rape may be a one off act.
- Most rape accounts will give an indication of violence. The after effects of sexual abuse including rape include psychological and social problems and stigma that the individual must learn to cope with among friends, colleagues and self and family members,
- Long-term effects of sexual abuse including rape are fear of men, aversion of sex, suspicion and lack of trust of men, depression, anger at men and resentment of men.

Identifying victims of sexual abuse

The teacher can help identify abused children and refer them to health personnel to be examined for the evidence of abuse where possible.

Abuse or rape is not an easy experience to talk about.

A teacher should be suspicious where:

- A child is withdrawn and depressed.
- The child may show a change in gait (walking style) he/she may limb as a result of the trauma and pain.
- A child is unable to pay attention to school tasks.
- A child may not show keenness to go home often hanging about a friend's place, or is just not in a hurry to go home.
- A child usually arrives at school very early but performs poorly in class.
- A child is not keen to get involved in school activities because of responsibilities at home.
- A child has poor faecal control and may regress in developmental milestones.
- An abused child, especially the young ones may display open sexual behaviours including masturbation.
- Some children may express anxiety about being left alone with a particular person.
- The child often has somatic complaints such as headache, stomach ache but displays extreme distrust and fear of being examined
- Children engaged in oral sex may have persistent sore throat due to sexually transmitted infections such as gonorrhoea
- The child may have an explicit knowledge of sexual behaviour, which may be displayed when playing with others or talking with others.

Refer the child to health personnel who will examine the child to confirm or dispel the suspicion.

Early marriages

Early marriages occur in some cultures where girls in particular are married off to elderly men before full developmental potential. Early marriages may be arranged for the following reasons:

- As a cultural practices
- As a pay off for debts
- In exchange for food in famine hit societies
- To avenge angry spirits of the wronged dead in some tribes.

- Some girls may fall pregnant with the first ovulation and before experiencing menarche and proceed to experience the trauma and complications of pregnancy and labour as children.

The school teacher must openly discuss this evil practice and encourage little girls subjected to this practice to report such practices. The school teacher can liaise with police or other human rights organizations to rescue the children.

Physical and mental abuse among children

Children can be subjected to physical and mental abuse in the societies in which they live. Abuse can be by parents or guardians. Children will not readily talk about this as they are often threatened with more punishment should they divulge the abuse. The teacher can identify cases of abuse through close observation of the child's behaviour at school.

A physically abused child may:

- Have bruises as a result of assault, or burns that the child may explain as accidents or any such difficult to believe explanation.
- Be unusually withdrawn
- Loses concentration in class
- Prefers to keep to herself instead of interacting with others.

Such children will open up to persons they trust. Cases of physical abuse must be reported to the police and social welfare or other humanitarian organizations with the welfare of children at heart.

Health Education

Children should be helped to limit the possibilities of abuse and rape.

- Children should be taught **never to allow** any person to touch their bodies or caress them.
- Children must be taught never to trust men, strangers and even relatives who can easily take advantage of them.
- Children must be taught to object to a man or woman touching their breasts, or any part of the body

- They must be advised to move away from the offender, and report to an adult or their parents.
- Children must be encouraged to have an open relationship with their parents to enable them to discuss intimate issues. If a young girl is invited for a date, she must discuss it with her mother or elder sister, take a friend with her or a bigger sister or brother.
- Young girls must be advised about the dangers of being **on their own with a man** in a dark places, a locked room or accept a car ride on their own
- Young girls **should not accept gifts from strangers** as the stranger may demand to be paid sexually.
- Young girls **should not accept a lift** in a car where they are alone with the driver or as the only girl. It is advisable for young girls to **always tell someone where they are going** and only go there if there is a good reason to be there.
- Children should also be informed of the dangers of **loitering** in the streets or in public places aimlessly as they can be taken advantage of and sexually abused.

Chapter 11

ADOLESCENCE (PUBERTY)

Adolescence is the stage of transition from childhood to adulthood. It is marked by a rapid physical growth and secondary development of sexual organs. This growth spurt may bring about a state of confusion in the young person because of the physical changes in the body. The upsurge of the growth hormones and sex hormones from the pituitary gland at the base of the skull brings about the changes transforming a young girl or boy into a young adult. From the age of eight years, little boys and girls begin to produce sex hormones in addition to the growth hormone. These sex hormones bring about significant changes in the growing child.

Changes in boys at Puberty

The sex hormone, Interstitial Cell Stimulating Hormone, and the increase in the Growth Hormone bring about the following changes in the young boy.

- There is an observable increase in height and development of muscle.
- The shoulders become broad.
- Boys will begin to grow a little hair on the chin which later becomes beard. Hair also grows in armpits and on the pubic area.
- The voice deepens, what is commonly referred to as breaking of voice.
- The reproductive system becomes fully developed with the genital organs increasing in size.
- The height of puberty in a young man is marked by maturation and full stimulation of the testicles to become active genital organs.
- Testicular tissue begins to produce the male seed, the **spermatozoa,** and **the hormone testosterone**, which causes maturation of the spermatozoa and is also responsible for sexual desire and further muscular development in the young man.
- Spermatozoa produced in the testicles swim in a white fluid, **semen,** which is also produced by the seminal vesicles and the prostate glands.
- Boys dream of erotic scenes and discharge semen with spermatozoa in their sleep, commonly referred to as **wet dreams**. Should a young man

have sexual intercourse from this stage of development and onwards, he is capable of becoming a father.

- There is the urge triggered by the sex hormone testosterone in the boy to experiment with the developed organs.
- The focus of the adolescent is on the fascinating developments on his body in particular the changes on the genital organs.
- It is important to note that young men have more difficulty controlling their hormones than girls do, hence the need for sexual health education around puberty.

Changes in girls

Changes in the female adolescent are driven by the rise in the Follicle Stimulating Hormone, which is very active together with the Growth Hormone. The increase in production of the hormones influences specific changes in specific body organs.

- The growth hormone influences the lengthening of bones and increase in size of all body organs.
- It is important to note that puberty does not come at the same time for all children of the same age. It may come as early as eight years in some children and may be as late as seventeen in others.
- During puberty, girls will observe a remarkable change in the breasts, which increase in size. They have a tingling itch as they grow especially at certain times of the month.
- The thighs and buttocks also increase in size, and the typical feminine curves begin to take shape.
- The female internal organs increase in size.
- The height of puberty in a young girl is menarche or menstruation, the beginning of monthly periods.

The Menstrual Cycle

The Follicle Stimulating Hormone (FSH) produced by the pituitary gland stimulates the ovaries(Llewelyn-Jones,1980). There are two ovaries in the female, but only one is stimulated each month.

- In the ovary are premature ova or eggs inside follicles or an equivalent of a nest. One of these follicles is stimulated to grow every month.
- The egg or ovum grows as the follicle grows. The follicular cells produce the hormone **oestrogen** in the first half of the month to cause significant monthly changes in the female internal organs.

Effects of oestrogen

- Oestrogen influences the uterus to grow and increase in size. The uterus develops an extra inner lining layer of tissue inside it.
- Oestrogen increases blood flow to the uterus and the pelvis as a whole causing a feeling of blotting and heaviness in the pelvis.
- Oestrogen causes thickening of blood and congestion in blood vessels causing tension headaches that result in irritability.
- Oestrogen changes mucus in the genital system especially in the cervix, to become thick.
- The vagina feels dry. The breasts fill up with fluid and become tense and itchy.
- The skin may become rough and dry. In some girls, pimples may appear on the face.

Leutinizing Hormone

Half way through the month, from about the eleventh day, small amounts of the hormone Leutinizing Hormone are produced by the anterior lobe of the pituitary gland.

- The Leutinizing hormone causes the ripening of the growing follicle in the ovary.
- small amounts of the hormone **progesterone** are produced by the cells of the follicle with the ovum ripens.

Effects of progesterone

- Progesterone causes an increase in blood supply to the uterus and increases the secretions in the female genital system.

- The increase in blood supply increases the typical feeling of congestion and discomfort women feel in the lower abdomen towards their periods.
- The mucus in the vagina becomes watery and slippery.
- During the stage of the flow of progesterone, the female body is highly stimulated and the desire for sexual intercourse is increased. If one has sexual intercourse, the thin watery mucus at this time of the month makes it easy for the spermatozoa to swim up the female genital tract.
- At around the fourteenth day from the start of the growth of the follicle, the ripe follicle opens releasing the mature ovum. This is called **ovulation.**
- The released **ovum** is directed into the fallopian tube by the finger like ends of the fallopian tube. It is further pushed towards the uterus by fine hairs called **cilia.**
- Inside the uterus, there is continued increase in thickness and blood supply in preparation for the arrival of the ovum.
- Should there be sexual intercourse at this stage, one is likely to fall pregnant because the released ovum is free and the female genital system is well prepared.
- The empty follicle produces what is called a yellow body or **corpus luteum**, which continues to produce progesterone. Should one have sexual intercourse, the ovum and the spermatozoon (one), will fuse in an event called **fertilization,** thus, one falls pregnant.
- If however, there is no fertilization, in about seven days after ovulation, the levels of progesterone in the body begin to decline as the corpus luteum dries off to form scar tissue.
- The thick internal layer of the uterus begins to disintegrate and comes out as blood through the vagina, in a process called **menstruation.** The extra blood that had collected in the uterus and the tissue that formed the extra layer, together with the ovum, are discharged out of the reproductive system as blood.
- It takes from three to five days for the blood to flow out. A few girls may bleed for seven days.
- The cycle repeats itself every month in a woman from puberty until the age of fifty-five years.

- As soon as a girl attains menarche, she must keep a record of her last normal menstrual period.

Period pains

Many young girls experience a lot of discomfort from a few days before the menstruation starts until the end of the menses. This discomfort comes at the peak of pelvic congestion due to increased blood supply to the reproductive organs especially the uterus.

- As degeneration of the inner layer of the uterus occurs, the uterus helps to expel blood through the cervix by contracting vigorously and rhythmically. **This is the major cause of the period pains.**
- The contraction affects all the organs in the pelvis that is the bowel, the bladder and pelvic muscles.
- Some girls may vomit; some may have a fast moving bowel while some may have an increased urge to pass urine. Others will experience a headache and a chill.

Managing Period Pain

The period discomfort may be eased by :

- Taking a *hot bath, or hot shower.*
- Placing a hot water bottle or warm compress over the lower abdomen to provide heat that relaxes blood vessels easing pain.
- Engaging in exercises especially, any sporting activities, sprinting, jogging, swimming, and any exercises that move the legs and pelvis such as sit ups and cycling will ease period pains.
- Some girls feel thirsty. It is wise to replace the lost fluid by drinking warm drinks, which also soothe the pain.
- Mild painkillers can be taken to relieve pain.

Feminine hygiene during menses

Young girls should be advised to:

- Keep clean during menses. It is possible to get infected during menses through the use of dirty or dusty cotton wool.
- Girls should be advised to use clean and hygienic sanitary towels.

- A clean sanitary towel must be worn every time on visiting the toilet and changed every two hours and when soaked. This prevents odours.
- Record the dates of menses to identify any abnormalities in the pattern of menses. A record of menses is useful should a girl experience problems with their menses later on, health personnel work with the date of the last normal period. The date is also required should one decide to use contraceptives and become sexually active.
- A record of menses enables assessment of risk of pregnancy in the event of sexual abuse.

Menarche is therefore a significant developmental stage and a major event and landmark in the female reproductive history.

Skin Changes

After puberty, the young person transforms into a young adult.

- The skin becomes very active.
- The body begins to sweat a lot especially where two skin surfaces meet, as well as in the palms.
- Sweat glands become very active too and a lot of body wastes are spilled out of the body through the skin.
- Sweat comes out in large amounts and is trapped in areas where two skin surfaces meet like the armpits, the elbows, the groins.
- Although the sweat cools the skin, after a while, the old sweat causes a nasty stale smell of the body.

Stale sweat and wastes must be removed from the surface of the body to keep the skin fresh and to keep the skin pores open. Adolescents must therefore be encouraged to take frequent baths.

- Just washing under the shower may not be good enough for some people with very strong body odors.
- Pubic and axillary hair remove be removed often. Long hairs in the armpits for example, trap the sweat in the armpits slowing its drying from the surface. The sweat may then soak into the clothes spreading the nasty smell and trapping it even further.

- Adolescents must be made to understand that it is not always easy to pick one's own nasty smell but a nasty smell draws everyone's attention.
- A nasty smell can also come from **sweaty feet** and **dirty socks** and **dirty underwear**
- Adolescents should be encouraged to **apply a deodorant** in the sweaty areas to control excessive sweating and to get rid of nasty smells. A deodorant does not have to be expensive. It is better to smell of a cheap deodorant than to smell of sweat.
- Encourage adolescents to wear clean socks and clean underwear every day. One should never wear socks twice before they are washed.
- Never sleep in their underwear them and wear them the next day. This is a source of a nasty smell.
- Large amounts of lubricating oil, **sebum**, is produced by the skin cells called **sebaceous glands** onto the skin surface. Some of this oil may be trapped in the secreting cells creating skin problems such as pimples and blackheads, resulting in rough skin and freckles on the face. Pimples make the skin appear rough and lumpy.
- Pimples can be quite distressing to a young person. Pimples are a phase of growing up. They eventually disappear from the face. It is **unwise to squeeze** pimples as squeezing causes swelling of other surrounding tissues and also leaves dark unsightly blemishes on the face.

Sexual Drive

- From menarche **every month, a young woman is likely to be ovulating every month and may fall pregnant** should they engage in unprotected sexual intercourse.
- There is a tendency for adolescents to start befriending fellow adolescents of the opposite sex. This is normal and natural. It is important that adolescents are made aware that having a friend of the opposite sex is normal and a part of growing up.
- The peer group may become an essential group for support for the adolescent and small subgroups with their group specific norms can be identified especially in a school set up.

- Crushes over girls or boys and even crushes over the school teacher, over older boys, and men, and for boys, over older girls and women may occur. **The adolescent of either sex can be taken advantage of sexually.**

- Sexual drive is intense at this stage because of the flow of sexual hormones. Teenagers can be assisted to think of alternative entertainment besides sexual activity. They must be encouraged to put their energies into developing and mastering a hobby that takes up much of their spare time and a lot of their energy.

- Adolescents should therefore be encouraged to participate in sports, joining the gymnasium to spend their energies on worthy causes. The school teacher should be innovative in introducing various sports so that the adolescents have a wide choice of sport at their disposal. When adolescents are engaged in competitive activity their energies are spent on the activities and their focus is drawn to activities and not their sexual drive. After sport or hard work and a cold shower, the sexual heat is usually subdued.

- Adolescents can engage in charity work like helping the vulnerable groups in society, the elderly, orphans and physically handicapped to fill up their spare time.

- Adolescents must be conversant with knowledge of sexual organs and how they function to give them a deeper understanding of how to avoid unwanted teenage pregnancy.

- Opportunities for an open discussion about sexual health must be available so that the adolescent is well informed. A school nurse or the local health centre nurse can be invited to provide accurate information in sexual health(Plummer et al;2006; Wight et al, 2002). Sexual desire is a basic instinct and should be openly discussed to guide the young and prevent sexual problems.

The teacher should however note that in some societies, sexual behaviour is according to the environment, and the culture of a given society. Patterns of sexual behaviour and norms are put in place by

society. For instance, among some African tribes, virginity is encouraged and on marriage, young women are expected to be virgins. Adolescents should have an opportunity to discuss such issues.

- Sexual health information should be available and accessible to all young adults so that they can make informed decisions about contraception, lifestyles, and choices.

- Sexual activity is a major step in a young person's life and has to be approached with full knowledge and responsibility of the consequences. Over eighty percent of young women fall pregnant without basic sexual knowledge and ninety percent of them without having used any family planning method. Many young women have to depend on the partner for sexual information; as a result, the ordinary young women maybe poorly informed and have misconceptions about sexual health(Murira et al.,2010)

- Parental guidance in sexual matters is strongly recommended and encouraged to inform the adolescent. Sexual information including information on healthy sexual life, fertility and family planning, problems encountered in sexual life such as sexually transmitted diseases including HIV/AIDS must be fully discussed and explained.

While **abstention** from sexual intercourse is the best way to keep out of the family way before one is ready for that responsibility, it is difficult for most adolescents to exercise control and restraint when aroused. It is also short-sighted for adults to expect adolescents to have total control over their sexual desire. It is therefore best that adolescents know how to prevent pregnancy.

- Inform adolescents that it is possible to say "NO" to sex and to keep one's word.

- It is best that adolescents are aware of safe sex, i.e. kissing, hugging, cuddling, deep patting, and use of protective methods to prevent disease and pregnancy.

- Adolescents should be advised on responsible sexual behaviour and learning to control oneself **to postpone the responsibilities that come with starting a family early,** and wait until one has achieved some basic goals in life, like securing somewhere to live independently, sustaining themselves financially, and having a faithful trustworthy partner.

- The advantages of preventing pregnancy by far out way the disadvantages of teenage pregnancy. It is unwise for young people to fall pregnant before they are ready for the responsibility of parenthood.

- Sexual intercourse without protection is a sure way to fall pregnant. Once sexual organs come into contact, it may not be easy to withstand the temptation to proceed and have sexual intercourse. Besides when a young man and young girl touch and caress and kiss, the genital organs are aroused and the female organs respond by becoming wet, which is a suitable environment for the male seed should it be released on the wet slippery environment. The male seed may easily swim up the female genital organs.

- In the male, semen with spermatozoa may start flowing through the male organs as soon as the male is excited and aroused by touching, kissing and caressing. Contact of the genital organs may cause a young man to ejaculate or release the semen prematurely especially that a young person has not yet learnt control and withholding. The result may be a quick sexual act with or without penetration but where semen is discharged onto the wet female organs resulting in a girl falling pregnant. It is best for adolescence to be aware of effective methods of family planning available that they can access easily.

Preventing Pregnancy

A girl or young man who admits that they are dating has a high chance of having sexual intercourse.

- The best and easiest method for prevention of pregnancy as well as sexually transmitted diseases is abstention but should there be failure to control the sexual urge, **a condom which prevents both sexually transmitted diseases and pregnancy <u>must be used.</u>**

- There are varieties of the pill, jellies and foams that young people who do not have regular sexual intercourse can use. While these may prevent pregnancy, they do not prevent sexually transmitted diseases including HIV/AIDS. It is therefore important for schools to liase with local health centre so that the methods of contraception available can be made known to those young adults who are sexually active or wish to be sexually active.

Teenage Pregnancy

Lack of information and poor guidance are increasingly causing adolescents as young as fourteen to indulge in unprotected sexual activity resulting in pregnancy and sexually transmitted diseases including HIV (Babalola et al.,2005). Pregnancy before a girl reaches the age of twenty is considered teenage pregnancy, although in many cultures the age of eighteen may be considered an age of maturity.

- Teenage pregnancy has many disadvantages, which must be avoided at all costs.
- Having a child requires a sound income.
- Babies are expensive, they require motherly love which means one is tied down with the chores of caring. Babies require clothes, food, which needs money.
- Babies fall ill, which requires caring skills and hospital bills.
- Indulging in sexual activity early in life exposes a young people to the risks of sexually transmitted diseases, pregnancy and pregnancy complications such as haemorrhage, infection, high blood pressure all of which are leading causes of maternal death(Sunmola et al.,2003).
- Indulging in sexual activity early in life predisposes to cancer of the cervix, the most common cancer in women.
- Early pregnancy means that one looses the opportunity to progress with education and settles for the family way and baby care duties.
- It is best to prevent unwanted unplanned pregnancy than to panic when one is pregnant and resorting to seek termination of pregnancy.

Abortion is not a family planning method. It is a desperate act to get rid of a pregnancy and is a very dangerous decision. Many young girls who

opt for abortion risk loosing their lives through heavy bleeding and infection after backyard abortions when they realise they can't be parents that early. Many women carry heavy guilty conscience after the abortions and live to regret throughout their lives. The young adolescent forfeits her opportunities for education.

Parenting is a full time job without pay and can lead to a cycle of poverty. **Baby dumping; giving away children for adoption all occur because young people have failed to handle their sexual responsibilities and realise that they cannot shoulder the responsibility of parenting. It is best to prevent unwanted pregnancy.**

Abnormal Sexual Behaviour

While some adolescents go through the stage of sexual development in a normal way, there are a few who display abnormal sexual behaviours that are worth reporting to health personnel so that the adolescent can receive the relevant advice and care.

Increased Libido

A high libido (sexual desire) is not uncommon in young adults but excessive libido in which an individual wants to have sex at any place and any time, and has insatiable desire for sex **(nymphomania)** is abnormal. This behavior is usually of psychological origin. Such an individual will need to be referred to a psychiatrist for counseling especially on measures of self-control.

References

1. Babalola,S; Tambashe, B.O; Vondrasek, C. Parental factors and sexual risk-taking among young people in Cote d'Ivoire. *African Journal of Reproductive Health*. 2005;9(1):123-128

2. Llewellyn-Jones, D. (1980) Fundamentals of Obstetrics and Gynaecology.Vol.11. Gynaecology. Faber and Faber

3. Murira,N; (2010) Communicating Sexual and Reproductive Health messages. Birmingham City University, Centre for Health and Social Care Research.

4. Plummer, M.L; Wight, D.Wamoyi, J et al., Are schools a good setting for adolescent sexual health promotion in rural Africa? A qualitative assessment from Tanzania. *Health Education Research*, 2006; 22 (4): 483-499

5. Sunmola, A.M; Dipeolu, M.; Babalola, S et al., Reproductive knowledge, Sexual behaviour and Contraceptive use among adolescents in Niger State of Nigeria. African Journal of Reproductive Health, 2003; 7(1):37-48

6. Wight, D; Raab, G.M; Henderson, M et al., Limits of teacher delivered sex education: Interim behavioural outcomes from randomised trials. *BMJ*, 2002; 324:1430

Chapter 12

SPORTS AND PLAY

Children naturally want to play and enjoy engaging in group activities and organized sport.

- A healthy child is active and is keen to discover things around him, experiment with things, and ask questions. The adage "All work and no play makes Johnny a dull boy," is true of children if the role of play in a child's life is to be considered.

- Play is the most important part of children' s time. The teacher must encourage children to play and participate in as many sporting activities as possible.

The importance of play

- Play is important for **improvement of general physical fitness**. As the children jump and hop about, they are exercising their bodies, burning up the stored fats and carbohydrates and strengthening their muscles

- Play is important for **movement of body joints** and prevention of rigidity that may cause bad posture and limited joint mobility.

- Exercise is important as a way of training the body to maintain **good body balance** and **coordination**.

- Activity **improves blood flow**, makes the heart to beat harder and faster pumping blood to all parts of the body and as the child runs about causing muscle and joint movement, blood flow to all parts of the body is improved.

- The hard breathing **draws in more air to the lungs**, which expand to the maximum. The fresh air is passed onto the blood as the blood gives off carbon dioxide from muscle activity. The fresh blood to the muscles prevents muscle cramps.

- **Exercise improves sleep**. After prolonged spells of play, children tend to enjoy a good sleep. A child who sleeps well wakes up refreshed and performs well in class.

- **Exercise improves appetite**. As the child plays and burns up stored energy, the body demands for food increase making the child's appetite to improve.

- Play **teaches the child patience, respect** for others and control of temper as the child learns to give others opportunities to take their turns at play and sometimes pick little quarrels that they resolve in their own manner or run to teachers for assistance.

- Play gives the child **a feeling of self- accomplishment** and **self-esteem** among peers. Organized group work **equips children with leadership skills** development and children want to lead as this increases their self-esteem. As new cognitive skills are incorporated into old skills this enhances skills and improves performance and competence and a child is motivated to do better than before.

- Many games **increase the concept of fairness** among children and **teach children to obey rules.**

- Games **promote the use of memory** when a child recalls how to play a game and this **develops logical reasoning**.

- Play is important for **improvement of language**. Play is necessary for **developing social skills** and cognitive activities and being with peers means that children can share common age specific language and skills.

- Some games have their specific language in the form of the rules of the game, cheering up or encouraging play, the declaration of winners and losers and the glory and esteem associated with good play.

- Through learning how to play a game, children's vocabulary improves. This explains why it is easier for children to learn new languages and new material. Teachers therefore should encourage play and should be able to notice a child who does not participate in play. Children may not play if they are not feeling well, if hungry, sleepy, or if the environment is not conducive for play such as where they are bullied.

Health Care Advice

- It is important to encourage children to participate in group and single activities and to support children's outside interests
- Parents must be encouraged to support children and praise children's successes to give a sense of self- worth. This is why it is necessary to invite them to attend school sporting activities.
- Parents must be encouraged to help children see their strength and weaknesses to strengthen their learning

Taking note of talent

- While some children may be good in academic subjects, some children may be good at sport. Children should be encouraged to excel in what they are good in and all the available assistance be given to assist a child do what they enjoy doing.

CHILD SAFETY

Accidents

Accidents are common in children with the causes of accidents varying according to the child's age.

Schools must take all the necessary measures to prevent accidents.
There are three factors that can be considered in accidents. These are, the agent, the host and the environment.

The agent

- Road traffic accidents, drowning, burns and fires are very serious accidents. Schools must put in place safety measures such as clear signposts for schools, entry gates, pedestrian entrance, exit gate and zebra crossing points for children to cross into the school premises and out of school. The zebra crossing must be manned at peak hours, that is in the mornings and when children finish school.

- Drop off areas must be clearly sign posted and ideally be off busy roads. The children must be taught street safety, crossing at designated places and bicycles riding rules.

- Simple agents tend to produce minor injuries. Simple injury may be caused by recreational equipment such as swings, bicycles, falls from heights, and during sports.

- Some accidents are associated with **the host**, meaning that the child herself is responsible for these with boys more prone to accidents than girls because boys tend to be more daring, play rough games, and want to show off in the presence of their colleagues.

The physical environment of the child can dictate the type and frequency of accidents a child may be exposed to.

- The social environment can expose the child to accidents. Children left to play unattended, are more prone to accidents compared to children whose activities are supervised.

- Over exposure of children to items that increase and expose them to accidents such as, pools, electricity, and firearms, matches, rivers, and dams should be avoided.

- Schools can work collaboratively with the local health authority to distribute pamphlets to educate communities on prevention of accidents in the homes, and environment.

- Safety of children is very important all the time. It is advisable to observe what children do and also listen to what children say.

- It is possible for some children to bring into the school items that may be harmful to others like knives, razor blades, screw drivers and guns. Parents must be encouraged to ensure that children are not in possession of such items and teachers too must be very observant.

- Some children may engage in dangerous games or as show off among peers and end up harming themselves or their peers.

- Grounds must be kept clean and level to prevent falls due to pits and ridges in the school grounds. Playground equipment should constantly be checked for fallen screws and tightening bolts

- Playfields must be free of items that may cause injury to children as they play.

- Equipment should be put away to avoid injuries. Any objects that are potentially dangerous must be reported.

Chapter 13

COMMON EMERGENCIES

Emergencies may arise at any time in schools because children are active and full of boundless energy. Children are curious and competitive and daring. Emergencies can arise as a result of circumstances beyond the control of the teachers or the children. In this chapter, brief advice on selected emergencies is given.

Emergency First Aid Kit

It is advisable that all schools keep an *Emergency First Aid Kit* where it is accessible to all members of staff.

This kit should preferably be contained in a box and the contents must be constantly checked and replaced after use.

An emergency kit should ideally contain:

Cotton wool roll,

Gauze swabs,

Gauze bandages,

Crepe/stretchy bandages of different sizes,

Triangular bandages for slings

A pair of scissors to cut bandages

Adhesive tape to secure bandages,

A mild antiseptic to wash the grazes

Glucose powder to make sweet drinks for anyone fainting during sports or because of hunger,

A small bottle of a mild analgesic e.g. panadol for mild pain like period pain,

A thermometer to check temperature where fever is suspected

Plastic gloves for handling injury

Safety pins to secure slings

Several packets of sanitary towels for emergencies.

- **A Sick Bay** or special side room should ideally be available at each school and equipped with a small folding bed and a blanket for emergencies.
- The telephone number of the **Ambulance**, the nearest **Doctor** or **health facility** should be written boldly on the wall and on the emergency box and inside the lid of the emergency box for everyone to see.
- Teachers should be trained in First Aid so that they can offer first aid services when emergencies occur in the school.

Bee Stings and Wasp stings

Some children react badly to stings and may go into shock (fainting, low blood pressure, rapid pulse, gasping for air.
- Lie the child in a recovery position and arrange to send the child to the nearest health centre.
- Sometimes bees and wasps leave their sting in the skin of its victim. These should be pulled out if possible but if one is not sure, call health personnel.

Precautions
- Children should be warned to move away from bees especially in the school flower garden
- Bee and wasp nests must be reported and the insects sprayed with an insecticide.

Bruises and Grazes
The First Aider must wear gloves before attending to bruises, graises, or bleeding.
- Clean water can be poured on the **graze** to remove grass and sand.
- Apply dry dressing or paint with antiseptic. Dressings should be available in the first aid box.

Cuts.
- Stop haemorrhage by padding with cotton wool and firm bandage and refer to health facility.

Bleeding from mouth
- Rinse the mouth with water and refer to health facility for assessment.
- Where bleeding is continuous, make a sizeable piece of cotton wool and place it against the bleeding sport.

- Let the child bite the cotton wool and keep it in place between the jaws to control haemorrhage until the child is seen by health personnel.
- Refer the child to the health facility immediately.

Nose Bleeding

- The tiny blood vessels inside the nostrils expand in hot whether and may burst causing nose bleeding (epistaxis).
- Some children may bleed because of very high temperatures and fevers.
- Some bleeding occurs in children with hereditary bleeding problems (**haemorrhagic diseases**).
- An accidental blow on the nose by objects like a football, or tennis ball can cause nose bleeding.
- A bad fall with face downwards may occur causing nose bleeding.
- The teacher must record the incident sighting what the child was doing before the bleeding, and whether the bleeding was spontaneous (starting without known obvious cause).

First Aid Measures

- Sit the child in a straight chair **with neck slightly extended to keep airways clear.**
- **Reassure the child.**
- Apply cold compress on forehead and change the compresses, as they get warm.
- Wash or wipe the child's face with a towel dipped in cold water.
- Advise the child not to blow nose.
- Observe for signs of swallowing which may mean that the child is bleeding and swallowing the blood.
- Check the pulse of the child every thirty minutes and record.
- If bleeding is heavy or uncontrollable, quickly refer the child to a health facility as soon as possible.

As a precaution:

- Children must be advised to wear hats all the time especially in hot weather.
- Children must be advised to play indoors or in the shed when the sun is very hot.

Fractures:

- Call ambulance immediately where possible.
- Control haemorrhage by padding open wounds then apply a firm bandage.
- **<u>Do not pull or try to straighten broken bone.</u>**
- Immobilize affected limb by tying both legs together if leg is broken.
- Pad a firm cardboard or plank in case of broken arm and put the arm against it.
- Apply a firm bandage tying both the plank/board and the broken arm.
- Transfer child to health facility as soon as possible
- Lift the child in one piece with as little movement of the affected limb as possible.

Foreign Body in Eye

- **W**ash eye with clean water.
- Discourage child from rubbing eye as the foreign body may be pushed deep into the eye structures cause more injury.
- If the object is sticking out do not pull it out as more damage can be caused.
- Do not blow into the eye.
- You can pad the eye with a clean eye pad and bandage lightly to prevent wind and dust .
- Send the child to a health facility as soon as possible.

Fainting.

- A child may faint because of hunger, because of high temperature, or because they are tired after a sprint on a sports day.

- Other causes of fainting could be low blood glucose due to conditions like diabetes.
- Whatever cause of the fainting, ensure there is free flowing air so that the child can breathe with relative ease.
- Prevent choking by lying child in a left lateral position with head extended. Offer a cold sweet drink to give energy.
- Depending on cause, allow child to rest to regain energy. If the fainting is due to hunger, a glucose drink may be given.
- Arrange for a meeting with parents and advise on providing adequate food for the child.
- If fainting is not due to exhaustion, arrange for child to be seen at health centre for further investigations.

Fires

Fires can cause loss of lives and property. It is important that every school has a fire policy and that risk assessment for fires is done every day .

Sources of fire

Uncontrolled burning, arson, wild veld fires, electrical fires, machines/cars, gases, ciggerettes

As a precaution:

- Ensure that there are no fires active or smouldering around school buildings or play fields. Children are curious and may push each other or fall into the fire sustaining extensive burns.
- All burning must be controlled and preferably done when there are no children in the school.
- If a fire must be lit, take precautions that the weather is calm and there are no strong winds blowing.
- Any fires must be lit at the furthest point away from buildings and the reach of children.
- Buildings must be constantly checked for loose and hanging electric wires which can cause sparks that can ignite buildings.
- Equipment in laboratories and kitchens must be regularly serviced.
- Electric sockets are best sealed with leads when not in use.

- Equipment should be switched off after use and plugs removed from sockets.
- There should be designated smoking areas where cigarette butts are collected in a safe container. Smoking in the classroom is highly dangerous because of the amount of paper and furniture in the classroom which can fuel a furious fire.
- A No Smoking Zone can be created in the school to keep the smoke and the possible risk of fires aware from pupils and colleagues. Smoking subjects pupils and other colleagues to passive smoke that is as bad as active smoking.
- Smoking damages the lungs, liver, heart and kidneys.
- **Smoking is habit forming and it kills.** Smoking must be discouraged.
- It is advisable for schools to have **fire drills** for the whole school at least once every term so that children and staff know what to do in case of fire.
- Schools must familiarise staff and children with the fire precautions so that when fire breaks out they follow the procedure they have been taught during the fire drill.
- Fire hydrants/extinguishers must be situated in strategic points in each classroom and special fire extinguishers for chemical fires must be available in laboratories.
- All members of staff and senior students must be taught how to use fire extinguishers in emergencies.
- It is advisable that classrooms, dormitories, function halls have emergency escape doors in case of fires, there must be alternate routes for children to escape buildings.
- Doors must not be blocked by furniture and other items.
- Doors to every building should have spare keys that are clearly labelled and kept where every teacher has access in case of emergency.
- Boarding houses must not be locked from outside at night.
- There must be escape doors clearly labelled in each building.

Active Fire

- In case of an active fire, the teachers should instruct children to be calm.
- A fire alarm must be sounded to warn everyone to vacate the building.
- The fire station must be summoned immediately.
- The teachers should steer away children from the source of fire as quickly and calmly as possible to a safe designated assembly point.
- Doors leading to the source of fire must be closed to keep flames contained and prevent wind from spreading the fire.
- A roll call of all the children should be taken and every child accounted for.
- The toilets and doors should be checked.
- Where the clothes of an individual catch fire and there is an active flame, roll child in a blanket.
- Should children's clothes catch fire, children should be taught <u>not to run</u> as this fuels the fire **but** to roll on the ground.
- Water can be poured on the person whose clothes have caught a live flame

Burns

Burns can be caused by electric fires, open fires, chemicals, and hot water. In the case of a child being burnt:

- Pour cold water on the burnt area or apply a cold compress to prevent blisters.
- Do not open the blisters.
- Send the child to health facility immediately.

Chemical burns.

- Laboratory chemicals cause chemical fires as children carry out experiments in the laboratories.
- Should a child sustain chemical burns, apply antidote immediately and send the child to the nearest health facility or doctor for further management.

As a precaution:

- Chemicals must always be safely locked away and only specific amounts needed for a particular experiment dispensed.
- Ensure that antidotes to commonly used chemicals are in stock and within reach but safely stored away.

- There should be adequate supervision of children and extra staff to supervise experiments.
- Disposal of chemicals must be controlled and supervised.

Drowning.

- Remove child from water.
- Ensure that the child is breathing.
- Lie on left lateral position with chin extended and one lower leg bent. Call for ambulance immediately.
- If not breathing start mouth-to-mouth resuscitation.

As a precaution:

- There should be a fence around the swimming pool and preferably the pool must be covered with a net when not in use and supervised all the time by persons who can swim and are trained in first aid.
- There should be a gate to the pool that is locked at all times and only unlocked by a member of staff when it is time for swimming.
- Swimming must always be supervised. Children should only be allowed in the pool when under supervision.
- It is not wise for one member of staff to allow several pupils into water, as she may not cope with emergencies. There should always be several lifesavers all the time moving around and focused on activities in the pool.
- Too many children in the pool make it difficult to pay attention to each child. Children must be given turns, a few at a time.
- Beginners need more attention and assistance in the pool.

Also refer to available First Aid Books

Chapter 13

Social Deviance

While there are acceptable rules and regulations in families and social structures and civil rules for the general public, there are certain individuals and groups in society who may decide to be defiant to the societal norms for several reasons. Young people may succumb to peer pressure. Deviant behaviours could be used to revenge society for scores an individual feels he has to settle against society. Some of these deviants may have a history behind them such as a broken home, orphanage, and failure or inability to apply oneself and achieve success.

Some deviants feel let down by families and society in general. Some resort to deviance in order to be noticed especially if they feel overshadowed by siblings or better achievers. Deviants will want to form a cult of their own and are happy to win followers. Deviants may engage in weird behaviours because they are too lazy to follow the accepted rules, they are stubborn and some may behave absurdly because they genuinely do not know the correct way to behave.

Most deviant behaviours start at puberty when one seeks social belonging and aspires to find an identity to himself. The teacher is best placed to identify deviant behaviours displayed by adolescents. Some deviant behaviours may persist into adulthood if they are not controlled early. The teacher should refer such a child to a psychologist and health personnel for help should a child display deviant behaviours. A few deviant behaviours are briefly discussed below.

Homosexuality

This is a situation in which an individual prefers to befriend and have sexual relationships with a partner of the same sex. A man who prefers sexual relationships with another man is gay, whereas a woman who prefers to have sexual relationships with another woman is lesbian and the cult is homosexual as opposed to heterosexuals in whom sexual relationships are between a man and a woman. This type of sexual behaviour is associated with upbringing and lack of trust of the opposite sex.

- Exposure of a young girl to paternal cruelty may make her feel safer with only those of her own sex.

- Early exposure of children to the sexual act confuses them and may lead to abnormal sexual behaviours. Children exposed to sexual act may imitate sexual act when they play, may draw diagrams of what they see, may use sexual language and may touch others inappropriately If the teacher suspects that children are exposed to sexual activities where they see the act in adults, the teacher should ask to talk to the child's relative or contact social services that can make arrangements to remove the child from such an environment.

- Sharing a bed should be discouraged in adolescents as this is likely to lead to trying homosexual/lesbian activities. Homosexuality is more likely to occur at puberty due to the influx of sexual hormones, and the resultant identity confusion that may occur in a young adult causing the young adult to adopt a psychological gender in which an individual believes she/he is who she/he is not.

- A school teacher should look out for adolescents with homosexual/lesbian tendencies who may befriend each other in an unusually intimate manner, touch each other on erotic areas, caress each other and show tendencies of homosexuality in the form of walking style, dressing, gestures, and imitating tone of voices of the opposite sex and advise.

Beastiality

Beastiality is abnormal sexual behavior in which a person has sexual intercourse with an animal. This behavior is known to occur among young people where an individual is shy to express feelings to the opposite sex and where one has poor control of their feelings. The behavior is weird and punishable by law. Adolescents should be warned about peer pressure to engage in abnormal sexual behaviours. Human beings should seek sexual relationships with other human beings and not with animals.

Substance Abuse

This is the use of harmful and intoxicating illicit substances such as alcohol, cannabis, weed, barbiturates and narcotics or drugs of addiction. Illicit drugs can be injectables, tablets or sniffing substances like glue, petrol, paint, powders, drinking any intoxicating substances, and smoking intoxicating weeds that produce a state of euphoria.

- This can be a big problem depending on where one lives, the friends and availability of the substances.

- As children grow and search for identity and belonging, they may be tempted to try all kinds of entertainments, experiments and behaviours to attract attention, recognition and just to be different and create their own image and identity.

- Some young people may be into trying body-enhancing substances to build muscles and portray a picture of strength, or look like certain characters that they have seen on television, on adverts, in papers or that they have heard of.

- Sport loving young adults may try all sorts of substances to enhance their performances and become famous.

- It is more likely that adolescents engaging in substance abuse may also engage in deviant behaviours to imitate friends and may team up with friends for the sake of belonging and fear of loosing friends.

- Drugs of any type especially those that give a false feeling of happiness and feeling high can be dangerous as they affect the brain of the individual, their character and behaviour. Such drugs become addictive so that one fails to function normally or live without them.

Identifying Substance abusers

- Persons using illicit substances can easily be noticeable as they may have mood swings of great excitement when they have a high concentration of the drug in their system.

- They may have an abnormal glare into space; red, protruding eyeballs, may salivate excessively and or may have a slur in their speech.
- Some may laugh incessantly and become a nuisance.
- Some get a feeling of being invincible and fearless and would like to show off this new feeling by being violent.
- Some engage in morally unacceptable behaviours like committing rape, sodomy, becoming a public nuisance.
- Some may engage in dangerous feats like jumping from heights, buildings or into waters of any depth. This happens because they loose a sense of reasonable thinking.
- Most usually neglect their personal hygiene becoming scruffy in outlook.
- Most people on illicit drugs have abnormal appetite, may display abnormal power, may become irrational, and may become restless and agitated or get into very deep sleep as the drug wears out.

The Risk of Substance Abuse
- Once there is suspicion of drug abuse in a child, it has to be investigated thoroughly and the child referred to health personnel for assistance.
- Continued use of drugs may result in involvement in crime of varied magnitudes especially when one is high, mental health illness and addiction.
- Once one is addicted, they usually are affected in their work and social life. They fail to secure jobs or keep jobs, and usually end up in institutions.
- Children need guidance on what is good and what is deplored by society, what makes one famous, and how to get there.
- Children especially adolescents need to be guided on healthy behaviours to emulate and to stay on the right side of the law.
- Drug abuse can be corrected through special clinics with psychologists and psychiatrists. Report drug abusers to health personnel as quickly as possible so that the individual can be assisted.

Chapter 15

High School Leavers and College Students

Young people's behaviour seems to be the same across economic, education and geographic divides. Such observations point at a general lack of sexual information and support among adolescents at a time young people are sexually active, suggesting that that young people act spontaneously under the strong urge of the sexual hormones and are unaware of safe sexual behaviours and sexual risks.

Socio-demographic factors such as age, education and place of residence have been observed to influence preconception sexual behavior (Ajzen, 1980;Maria, 2006; Macintyre et al., 2006) suggesting that behaviour unfolds within a context influenced by social norms and beliefs. Reckless sexual behaviours among youths have been associated with lack of sexual health information suggesting the need to educate youth to increase perception of preconception risk (Wagbatsoma & Okojie, 2006).

Sex education should not therefore be left to health personnel only because health personnel see women after they are already sexually active. Without sexual education at home, in schools, youth centres, church groups and social clubs and wherever young people frequent or come together, there will be limited messages to the young people about safe sexual behaviours. These messages should include creation of awareness of contraception and prevention of sexually transmitted diseases.

There are three parental factors that have been identified as having a great influence on youth sexual behavior. The factors are; living with a father in the household during childhood, perceived parental disapproval of early pregnancy, and open parent-child communication about sexual behavior (Babalola et al., 2005). Parental communication with their adolescent children is emphasized and recommended as re-enforcing positive sexual behaviours, but research has also revealed that most parents are embarrassed, uncomfortable and lack skills to communicate sexual information to their children. Links between schools, parent education and health personnel can assist the parents to deliver sexual health messages to their adolescent children (Turnbull et al., (2008).

Teachers can get special training in sexual education to increase young people's knowledge of sexual and reproductive knowledge (Iyoke et al., 2006). Multiple interventions of teacher and peer education strategies have been found to improve knowledge, attitudes and self-efficacy in the sexual and reproductive health of students (Ajuwon & Brieger (2007).

There is consensus among researchers that lack of standardised sexual health education in schools, and a lack of parental teaching and guidance of adolescents is largely to blame for careless sexual behaviours among young people(Wagbatsoma & Okojie, 2006; Ajuwon & Brieger, 2007; Babalola et al., 2007; Turnbull et al., 2008; Lema et al, 2008; Reeves et al,2006). Sex education is uncommon in many schools even in the developed world resulting in women approaching their first pregnancies without the relevant amount of sexual and reproductive information (Plummer et al., 2006).

Some suggested strategies to confront barriers to contraception are working with community leaders, emphasizing the use of condoms as the only method with a dual action of preventing both pregnancy and HIV and use of multiple information sources for young people such as word of mouth, radio, leaflets, magazines, internet (Keele et al.,2005; Kankasa et al.,2005; Bankole et al.,2007).

Sexual health education alone may not suffice in reducing teenage pregnancy; but addressing some aspects of culture, development of young people's economic independence that empower the women to be self - sufficient and self determinant on when they may decide to fall pregnant, may delay pregnancy in young women.

While the adolescent is excited and sometimes impatient to reach adulthood, it is important for the young adult to be reminded that the next stage in development is the most demanding. Decisions that may influence the rest of one's life have to be made. There is need for attention to details that seem unimportant or were previously unknown. There is a gradual increase on the load of responsibilities one is expected to shoulder by virtue of being an adult. There is a demand on the attainment and maintenance of the highest quality of well being for one to survive the physical, social and psychological demands of adulthood.

Research has revealed that there is a collection of concepts and facets; inner circle specific feminine knowledge, attitudes, beliefs, values, taboos, behaviours, practices and duties, rules expected of women in a particular culture from the pre-conception period onwards. It is this collection of concepts and facets that differentiates the two genders into male and female. Gender specific knowledge and practices distinguish feminine behaviours from masculine behaviours (MacLauchgan, (2004). The women's culture is bound by shared local beliefs, attitudes and values derived from community interaction which is the source of knowledge and community ethos.

Understanding the women's culture and their health beliefs is the basis for understanding the women's attitudes, their intentions and the focus of their health behaviours (Airhihenbuwa,2004). It is important for the school teacher to have cultural understanding of the communities from which his/her learners come. Such information is essential in articulating health messages and ensuring that the health messages are well received and do not offend communities and families.

The importance of good health and being able to maintain it at this stage of development cannot be overemphasized. Below are a few areas of health that a young adult needs to pay attention to at this stage of development along the lifeline.

Reference

1. Airhihenbuwa C.O. and Webster, J.D. (2004) Culture and African contexts of HIV/AIDS prevention, care and support. *Journal of Social Aspects of HIV/AIDS Research Alliance.* 1(1), pp. 4-13.

2. Ajzen,I; Fishbein,M)*Understanding attitudes and predicting social behaviour.* Englewood Cliffs,1980. NJ: Prentice Hall

3. Ajuwon,A.J; Brieger,W.R. Evaluation of a school-based Reproductive Health Education programme in rural South Western, Nigeria. *African Journal of Reproductive Health,* 2007;11(2):47-59

4. Babalola,S; Tambashe, B.O; Vondrasek, C. Parental factors and sexual risk-taking among young people in Cote d'Ivoire. *African Journal of Reproductive Health.* 2005;9(1):123-128

5. Bankole,A; Biddlecom,A;Guiella,G. et al., Sexual Behaviour, Knowledge and Information Sources of Very Young Adolescents in Four Sub-Saharan African Countries. *African Journal of Reproductive Health,* 2007; 11 (3) : 99-105

6. Iyoke,C.A; Onah,H.E; Onwasigwe,C.N. Teachers' Attitude is not an impediment to Adolescent Sexuality Education in Enugu, Nigeria. *African Journal of Reproductive Health,* 2006; 10 (1): 81-90

7. Kankasa,C; Siwale,M; Kasolo F et al., Socioeconomic and reproductive factors associated with condom use within and outside of marriage among urban pregnant women in Zambia. *African Journal of Reproductive Health,* 2005; 9 (3):128-136

8. Keele,J.J; Forste,R; Flake,D,F. Hearing Native Voices: contraceptive use in Matemwe village, East Africa. *African Journal of Reproductive Health,* 2005;9 (1): 45-49

9. Lema, L.A., Katapa, R.S. and Musa, A.S. (2008). Knowledge of HIV/AIDS and sexual behaviour among youths in Kibaha District, Tanzania. *Tanzania Journal of Health Research.* 10(2), pp. 79-83.

10. Macintyre,S; McKay,L; Ellaway,A. Lay concepts of the relative importance of different influences on health; are there major socio-demographic variations? *Health Education Research Theory and Practice*, 2006; 21 (5):731-736

11. MacLachlan, M. *Culture and Health.* A Critical Perspective towards Global Health. 2nd Ed. John Wiley & Sons Ltd. 2006.Chichester.

12. Maria, W. (2006). Sexual Behaviour, Knowledge and Awareness of Related Reproductive Health Issues among Single Youth in Ethiopia. *African Journal of Reproductive Health.* 10(3), pp. 45-50.

13. Plummer, M.L., Wight, D., Wamoyi, J., Nyalali, K., Ingall, T., Mshana, G., Shigongo, Z.S., Obasi, A.I. and Ross, D.A. (2006). Are schools a good setting for adolescent sexual health promotion in rural Africa? A qualitative assessment from Tanzania. *Health Education Research.* 22(4), pp. 483-499.

14. Reeves, C., Whitaker, R., Parsonage, R.K., Robinson, C.A., Swale, K. and Bayley, L. (2006). Sexual Health Services and Education: Young people's experiences and preferences. *Health Education.* 65(4), pp. 368-379.

15. Turnbull, T; Wersch, A. Van Schaik. A review of parental involvement in sex education: The role for effective communication in British families. *Health Education Journal,* 2008: 67 (3):182-195

16. Wagbatsoma, V.A; Okojie, O.H. Knowledge of HIV/AIDS and Sexual Practices among Adolescents in Benin City Nigeria. *African Journal of Reproductive Health,* 2006; 10: (2) 76-83

Chapter 13

SEXUALLY TRANSMITTED INFECTIONS (STI'S)

These are diseases that are contracted through engaging in sexual intercourse without protection (Merck Manual,2006). Sexually transmitted diseases include gonorrhoea, Chlamydia, syphilis, trichomoniasis and HIV.

Sexually transmitted infections (STIs) are caused by:

- Bacteria
- Viral pathogens
- Fungal pathogens
- Protozoan pathogens

CHLAMYDIA INFECTION

- This infection is now the most common of all bacterial STIs.

Symptoms and Signs

Many infected people may however have few or no symptoms of infection.

- Chlamydia infection may cause a thin watery genital discharge
- One may have burning sensation on passing urine (dysuria).
- In women chlamydia causes pain on sexual intercourse (dyspareunia).
- Chlamydia infection causes blockage of fallopian tubes in women causing ectopic pregnancy and infertility.
- In men Chlamydia causes swelling of testes (orchitis

Complications

- Chlamydia infection causes swelling and blockage of the vas deference, the tube that carries sperm from testes into the genital organs (epidydimitis).)
- Swelling of testes which may cause low production of spermatozoa,
- Blockage of the epidydimus causes male infertility.
- In women Chlamydia infection may lead to pelvic inflammatory disease (PID), one of the most common causes of pain in the pelvis
- Blockage of Fallopian tubes as healing occurs causes ectopic pregnancy and infertility.

Treatment

- One must report the above symptoms to health personnel.
- Take the full course of medication.
- Drink a lot of fluids to wash away infection from the urinary system.

Prevention

- Have one faithful sexual partner
- Use a condom always
- Wash the genital area thoroughly with soap and water twice daily and after sexual intercourse.

GENITAL HERPES

Genital herpes is caused by herpes simplex virus (HSV).

Symptoms and Signs

The infected person may feel a tingling or burning sensation in the groins, buttocks, and genital region.

- The major symptoms of herpes infection are painful blisters that open to become weepy sores.
- The sores may become infected and look dirty with patches of pus.
- The herpes sores usually disappear within two to three weeks.

Treatment

- Suppressive antiviral therapy can be used to prevent occurrences but these antiviral drugs do not destroy the virus.
- The sores can be washed and painted with antiseptics.

Complications

- The virus remains in the body for life and the blisters and sores may recur from time to time.
- Genital herpes can be transmitted to newborn babies during childbirth. Untreated HSV infection in newborns can result in mental retardation and death.
- One has high chances of contracting other sexually transmitted infections including HIV

Prevention

- Have one sexual partner

- Use a condom
- Wash the genital area thoroughly after sexual intercourse using soap and water

SYPHILIS

- Syphilis is a curable sexually transmitted infection caused by the bacteria **Treponema pallidum**

Symptoms and signs

- Early symptoms of syphilis may go undetected because they are very mild and disappear spontaneously.
- The initial symptom is usually **a painless open sore** with raised margins that appears on soft tissue such as the penis, the vagina, lips, and gums, under the nails and around the anus.
- The second stage of syphilis is marked by a transient rash on the face, the neck and may spread to the whole body.
- In its advanced stages syphilis causes large open wounds especially on the legs (gammatous lesions).

Treatment

Syphilis can be successfully treated with antibiotics.

- One must report any of the above symptoms to health personnel as soon as they are aware of them.
- One should have their sexual partners treated as well and must take the full course of antibiotics.

Complications

- Syphilitic heart disease can occur
- The brain and nervous system can be affected. One can have mental instability and poor balance and paralysis
- Syphilis is a major cause of abortions, stillbirth and death of the newborn babies

Prevention of syphilis

- Abstention from early sexual activity is the best and most effective way of preventing sexually transmitted infections. Young people must be encouraged to delay sexual relations for as long as possible.
- Any sexually active person must have a sexual relationship with one uninfected partner. It is important to go for tests before having sexual contact with a new partner. If one has a one night stand, one <u>must use a condom.</u>
- A condom should be used correctly and consistently and not selectively or occasionally!
- Sexually active people must be encouraged to prevent and control other STIs to decrease possibility of HIV infection and to reduce other infections if one is HIV-infected.
- The risk of acquiring STIs increases with the <u>number of partners over a lifetime.</u>
- Once one has been diagnosed with STI's, it is important to notify all recent sex partners and urge them to get a check up.

Treatment
- Syphilis can be treated with antibiotics
- The doctor's orders must be followed and one should complete the full course of medication prescribed to eradicate the infection.
- When one is on treatment, they should avoid all sexual activity and consumption of alcohol.
- A follow-up test to ensure that the infection has been cured is often an important step in treatment.

GENITAL WARTS
- Genital warts are caused by **human papilloma virus** (HPV), a virus related to the virus that causes common skin warts.

Symptoms:

Genital warts usually first appear as small, hard painless bumps in the vaginal area, on the penis, or around the anus.

Treatment
- Genital warts are treated with a drug applied to the skin or

- by application of extremely cold rods (freezing) which stops their growth and spread.
- If the warts are very large, they can be removed by burning them, (cauterization).

Complications

- If untreated, the genital warts may grow and develop into a fleshy, painless cauliflower-like appearance that may make sexual intercourse impossible.
- Certain high-risk types of HPV are thought to cause cancer of the cervix, the uterus, and other genital organs.

Prevention

- One must have one faithful sexual partner
- One must use a condom all the time

GONORRHOEA

This is a sexually transmitted infection by gonococci bacteria.

Symptoms and signs

- A person with gonorrhoea discharges **pus** from the vagina or penis
- One feels pain or difficulty in passing urine (dysuria).
- One can have abscesses in the groins in both men and women (bubos) in between the labia in women (Bartholinitis) and around the anus (peri-anal abscesses).

Treatment

- Gonorrhoea is treated with antibiotics.
- One should take the full course of antibiotics and one's sexual partners must also be treated.
- One should wash the genital area with soap and water at least twice a day.
- One must take plenty of oral fluids and avoid alcohol.

Complications

- It is important that one seeks help early from health professionals before serious complications occur.

- Gonorrhoea causes blockage of free flow of semen and spermatozoa from the testes. Male infertility can occur.
- Blockage of fallopian tubes by pus causing the uterine tubes to narrow or be completely closed. In women blockage of the fallopian tubes by gonococci infection is a major cause of ectopic pregnancy (pregnancy in the tubes outside the uterus).
- In men gonococcal infection causes swelling of the testes (orchitis), which interferes with production of spermatozoa, the male seed, causing a low sperm count and defective sperms.
- Gonococcal infection can be transmitted to a newborn baby at birth causing sore, pussy eyes (gonococcal opthalmia neonatorum).
- Gonococcal tonsilitis can occur in those who practice oral sex.
- Infertility in both men and women. Gonococcal infection in men may cause blockage of the vas deference, the tube that transmits sperm from the testes. Completely closed tubes prevent the female egg from meeting the male seed resulting in infertility.

Prevention
- Have one sexual partner.
- Use a condom always.
- Wash thoroughly with soap and water after sexual intercourse

TRICHOMONAS VAGINALIS
Tichomonas vaginalis infects both male and female genital organs.
- Trichomoniasis, causes a nasty, greenish, itchy, fishy- smelling watery vaginal and penile discharge. This causes irritation and soreness. One feels like scratching the genital area every now and then.

Management
- One needs very high standards of hygiene. Wash twice daily to remove sweat, wash away the smelly discharge and reduce the odour. Wear clean underwear.
- Drink plenty of fluids to reduce urinary tract irritation.
- Trichomoniasis can be treated. The sexual partner(s) must be treated too.

- Abstain from intercourse while on treatment and commence sexual activity when sure that the infection is clear.

Prevention
- Use clean pads that are changed regularly when having menses.
- Stick to one sexual partner
- Use a condom.

Complications of Trichomonas Vaginalis Infection
- In females it causes swelling of the vagina tract (vaginitis) causing pain on intercourse(dyspareunia)
- Trichomonas Vaginalis causes swelling of the urinary tube from the bladder, (urethritis) and swelling of the bladder (cystitis), resulting in pain when passing urine (dysuria) in both men and women.
- Trichomoniasis causes pain in the pelvis (pelvic inflammatory disease or PID)
- Scars when healing can cause ectopic pregnancy and infertility.

GENITAL CANDIDIASIS(Thrush)

This is infection of the genital organs by yeast called **Candida albicans.**

Symptoms and signs
- In men candidacies causes swelling of the urethra resulting in heat and pain when passing urine.
- There maybe a slight discharge, reddish and white patches on the glans penis and under the foreskin.
- There is swelling of the top or head of penis (glands penis) and irritation and soreness of the glans penis especially after sexual intercourse.
- Vulval irritation that makes the genital area reddish and swollen
- The vaginal wall is usually coated with a white milk curd-like substance which may bleed or leave a raw, red patch when removed.
- An offensive vaginal discharge is common in women.

Target population infected

- Persons with multiple sexual partners
- Persons who have had prolonged use of antibiotics
- Pregnant women
- People with diabetes
- People with anaemias.
- People with immune-suppressive syndromes and taking steroids.

Management

- In females Candidiasis causes swelling of the vaginal tract (vaginitis) and swelling of the external female genital organs (vulvitis). These body parts must be carefully washed with soap and water at least twice a day.
- Candida albicans can be treated and responds well to antifungal creams and pessaries.

Complications

- In severe cases there maybe swelling of the foreskin causing the skin to swell tightly around the glands penis (Phimosis) or crack and roll backwards (paraphimosis).
- Circumcision will be needed to correct this very painful condition.

Male Circumcision

Male circumcision is the surgical removal of the foreskin in men.
Circumcision does not prevent sexually transmitted diseases but limits infection by at least 60%.

- Where there is a foreskin micro-organisms hide and multiply under the skin fold.
- Surgery removes the harbour and makes the skin tough and easy to wash. One can still be infected through bruising during sexual contact.

HIV Infection

- Young people must be aware of the simple signs of HIV infection in any man who approaches them or a young woman one may fancy.

- Any young man/woman who catches flues, chills, coughs and sore throats every now and then and suffers from fevers even in the dry heat of the hot seasons is suspicious.
- Thrush in the mouth of an adult should be suspect.
- Swollen lymph nodes behind the ears are signs of infection.

Prevention
- Take time to know your partner.
- Use a condom. Unprotected sex exposes one to the diseases
- **Go For An HIV Test** when you think you are in love and before you have an unprotected sexual activity!
- Teenagers should avoid older sexual partners who are looking for a sexual relationship and not love. They have seen and collected it all and are likely to pass on sexually transmitted diseases to an unsuspecting partner.

Complications
- Repeated sexually transmitted infections may cause collection of pus in parts of the pelvis causing pelvic abscesses.
- Pus may block fallopian tubes resulting in failure to have children in future (sterility).
- One may progress to develop Acquired Immune Deficiency Syndrome

Young children and HIV/AIDS

Children have a very high chance of being born infected if one of their parents is infected by the virus! HIV positive children do grow up to reach school going age and proceed to adulthood.

- Some may not show any ill health until the ages of eight or above.
- Other children may have a poor health and may often be absent from school due to ill health. Such children usually look sickly and fail to grow at the expected rate of growth for their age.
- HIV positive children may have rough skin and are prone to skin diseases like boils and ringworm.
- HIV positive children are prone to repeated tonsillitis and chest infections.

- They usually have enlarged glands that are prominent between the angles of the jaw and neck.
- The school teacher should be able to identify a sickly child and get to know their underlying health condition. Knowledge of a child's diagnosis helps the teacher to quickly call for help in case of emergency or refer the child to the nearest clinic/health facility. It also helps the teacher to take the necessary precautions to protect other children.

Causes of HIV/AIDS in Adolescents

Culture

- In some families, young girls are expected to take over a sister's husband or an aunt's husband after the death of a sister or an aunt. Advise children and young people to refuse to be involved in such cultural practices
- Advise adolescents to refuse to be involved in such cultural and inheritance practices which predispose them to HIV/AIDS.
- Advise young girls to refuse to be married off to old men in the society for whatever reason, economic, religious or cultural.
- Advise children to report child abuse to someone they trust like the church minister or police because this is and exposes them to sexually transmitted diseases including HIV.

Beliefs

- Some men and women think smart looking partners cannot have STDs.
- Some people are just careless and will not take precautions
- Some men and women believe that they can cleanse themselves of the HIV through sexual intercourse with young children.
- Young adults must report any attempts to abuse them as it leads them to contracting STIs

Unprotected Sexual intercourse

HIV in Adults is spread through sexual intercourse between men and women or between men in homosexual relationships. Demand that your partner have an HIV test before having sexual intercourse.

- Once one is infected, one's sexual partner will most likely be infected too.
- It may take years, from two years to ten years before one feels unwell depending on how strong the infecting virus is and how healthy the infected individual is.
- An infected person who has not yet developed the disease may look well and have no symptoms. The presence of the virus can be detected through a laboratory test and quick tests done by health institutions.
- Once an individual has the virus in their system, it does not go away because **drugs known to date cannot kill the virus**.

Previous Sexually Transmitted Infection
- Adults infected by the virus will usually or may have experienced other sexually transmitted diseases like thrush of the genitals, genital warts, boils in the groins and the genital parts, genital sores and genital discharge of varying types such as the thick creamy pus of gonorrhoea usually combined with syphilis.
- Urinary tract infection characterized by lower abdominal pain and discomfort and pain on passing urine is also common.
- A few people may be deceived by the fact that they may not have suffered any of the sexually transmitted diseases and may therefore have a false feeling of wellness.

Signs and Symptoms of AIDS
The human immune- virus **weakens the body's ability to withstand diseases**. The body fails to protect itself against minor health problems that in normal circumstances would have been easy to deal with. All systems of the body are affected and one is very ill.

The initial stages of the presence of disease, AIDS, may present like flue. One feels weak, feverish, and feels hot and cold. One may have a headache.

- There is profuse sweating at night and a general feeling of ill health. These symptoms may repeat themselves several times and quite frequently.
- As the illness progresses, the blood **falls short of its major components** like iron resulting in a person looking pale, breathless and weak and frail.
- All the systems of the body are affected.

The Skin

- The **skin becomes rough**. A stubborn rash may occur on the face and body. Some people may develop a skin disease of one type or another, the most common being **Herpes** that may appear on any part of the body as a dense weepy painful rash that dries off after a week and almost always leaves behind ugly scarred tissue. This is a typical skin reaction due to the viral poison.
- Boils may occur on any part of the body.
- Wounds fail to heal.
- The hair becomes thin, straight and unhealthy like that of a malnourished child.

The Circulatory System

- The **heart is weakened**. One feels breathless at slight effort. The blood flow is affected and feet swell.
- If **bleeding occurs, such as in minor injury, surgery, and tooth extraction, it becomes very difficult to control.**
- The teacher must ensure that bruises and grazes and bleeding as the children play must be managed with caution. Use gloves always when handling injuries to prevent infection from infected blood. Other children must desist from handling blood with bare hands and must be made

aware of the precaution against cross infection and to call a teacher in case of injuries.

The Immune System

- Antibodies that protect against diseases cannot control these symptoms resulting in the body being attacked by any bacteria or virus that comes by, (**opportunistic infections**).

The Respiratory System

- **Bacterial infections** like **pneumonia and tuberculosis** occur repeatedly. These two conditions cause severe chest pain and breathlessness, and a persistent cough.
- The lungs may be filled with fluid preventing them from taking in oxygen and expanding as expected in the process of breathing.
- Drugs given to treat tuberculosis and pneumonia offer a temporary relief and do not completely heal the lungs, which remain with permanent scars and are likely to get re-infected.

The Digestive system

The digestive system is inflamed.

- The mouth may have a white coating (thrush), which is more marked in the morning when one wakes up. The lips become swollen and the skin peels off leaving blisters and raw flesh.
- The rest of the digestive system is swollen and irritable and fails to digest food or absorb it resulting in **indigestion and diarrhoea**, loss of appetite, vomiting and loss of weight.

The Brain

- The thin layer of tissue that covers the brain may become swollen, a condition known as **meningitis.**
- Meningitis causes severe persistent headaches and irritability.
- Meningitis may cause **mental confusion, blindness, loss of hearing, and stroke**.

- **AIDS has no cure**! Whatever drugs are circulating now, just give a temporary feeling of well being but do not kill the virus. No ancestral spirit , cultural ritual or religious prophets can remove the virus from one's body either, once one is infected!

- Every member of society has a responsibility to stop the spread of the virus haunting the societies and leaving behind untold suffering. AIDS is a long-term disease. One may suffer from ill health for many years before one succumbs to the disease. It affects work, and yet it is very expensive to live with the disease.

- One has to be seen regularly by the doctor and buy expensive drugs. One has to eat well too to keep healthy. A poor diet can only make one deteriorate faster.

- It is not necessary to suffer from this disease because it is preventable. A teenager can make her contribution towards prevention of the spread of AIDS in the following simple ways:

Advice to Teenagers:

Having a boyfriend/girlfriend is normal and is part of growing up; but, a boyfriend and girlfriend can see each other every day to talk and enjoy each other's company without indulging in sex.

- Young women especially must learn to say **"NO"** when it comes to sex. There is no hurry. Sex can be postponed. It is one activity, which will always be there for life.

- The teacher can help young adolescents set themselves objectives to achieve in life. The most important of these is to work hard at school and achieve good grades that will open doors to a much brighter future for them. Rushing to have sex may be a rush to contract HIV/AIDS

- The teacher must advise young adolescents against spoiling their chances of doing great things in life by indulging in sex early in life. There is so much to loose by indulging in sex at an early age and yet there is so much to gain when they postpone sex until they are mature, have a good job, have seen the world and are ready to deal with the demands of a sexual relationship.

Self-protection

- Teenagers must be careful not to be lured into sexual relationships with old and mature partners, no matter what they offer.

- Teenagers must avoid the macho man, or the popular girl who is dated by half a dozen men. It is best to have a partner that one has known for a while. A one night stand could have the virus. An HIV test before sexual contact could save one's life.

- Teenagers should not be cheated by looks. It is not easy to tell who has the virus just by looking at a person. By the time it is obvious, it is already too late for many who may have had sexual relationship with the individual.

- Teenagers must be advised that rushing to indulge in a sexual activity is a sign of poor self-control which can take one's life.

- The surest way for anyone to know if their partner is a safe sexual partner is to go for an **HIV Test** when they think they are in love!

There are suggestions to actively involve parents as participants and leaders in sexual health promotion in communicating sex related matters to their adolescent children (Airhihenbuwa & Webster, 2004; Marchant et al., 2004). Parental guidance on contraception should help the adolescents to make informed choices of contraceptive methods available (Mturi, 2003; Sunmola et al., 2003).

There are further suggestions that parents be the primary source of information on sex education as they are in a position to observe their adolescent children's development and behaviour. Other organizations like schools and the health system can complement parents messages with scientific information on foundations already laid down by the parents. But in many cultures, there is need to address the attitudes, and the values of the parents about sex education.

Sex is mystified and not openly talked about in many cultures. This attitude is currently a barrier to adolescent sex education in such countries.

Radio campaigns can be used to change the attitudes of the communities as first line teachers of adolescents as well as encouraging sex safe practices among the young people (Otoide, 2004; Lema et al.,2008).

While it is common knowledge that adolescents are at high risk of contracting HIV and other sexually transmitted infections, adolescent sex education is not provided for in schools in many countries especially in Africa (Plummer et al., 2006). The objective of sexual health information at this stage in life is to pass health messages about how the adolescents' bodies function to empower the young people with knowledge before they become sexually active so that they become competent in making informed sexual decisions (Reeves, 2006). Reports on adolescent sexual health education suggest that sexual knowledge among adolescents varies in content, teaching method, training of teachers and the level at which the sex education is introduced in school (Reeves et al., 2006).

Living with an infected person
- Many children may find themselves having to live with or look after members of the family suffering from HIV/AIDS. It is helpful if they have an idea of how to protect themselves from contracting the virus and how to help their loved ones who may be infected.
- If a child lives with someone suffering from Aids, he/she can encourage them to live as normal a life as possible. It is possible for them to live as normal a life as possible if they:

Follow the doctor's advice.
- Medicines prescribed must be taken as instructed.
- New health problems attended to as quickly as possible
- They must eat healthy food and three meals a day plus a snack in between meals.
- They must eat lots of fresh fruit and vegetables.

- They must avoid alcohol. It irritates the bowel
- They must be encouraged to stop smoking. Smoking weakens the lungs.
- They should keep high standards of hygiene to prevent skin infections.
- They must get themselves plenty of fresh air by taking walks early morning and evenings.

If the individual is very ill and needs caring:

Remember to wash your hands after handling them.

- Protect yourself from everything that comes from the body like urine faeces, sweat, and saliva. They must be well disposed of.
- Use gloves whenever you handle faeces and urine. In the absence of gloves, improvise with plastic bags.
- If one has an open wound, make sure it is securely bandaged.
- Wash clothes and bedclothes separately from other members of the family as these may have body fluids.
- If possible, soak clothes of the sick person in a bucket with a disinfectant for a while before washing them.
- Use separate utensils (cup, plate, spoon, fork, knife).
- Encourage them to clean the mouth regularly as it easily gets infected with thrush
- Give them frequent nutritious diet that is easy to digest like mashed foods, purees, soups, and fortified drinks.
- Encourage them to walk around to improve blood flow in the body.

References

1. Airhihenbuwa C.O. and Webster, J.D. (2004) Culture and African contexts of HIV/AIDS prevention, care and support. *Journal of Social Aspects of HIV/AIDS Research Alliance.* 1(1), pp. 4-13.
2. Lema, L.A; Katapa,R.S; Musa,A.SKnowledge of HIV/AIDS and sexual behaviour among youths in Kibaha District, Tanzania. *Tanzania Journal of Health Research,* 2008;10 (2):79-83
3. Merck Manual of Diagnosis and Therapy (2006) 18th Ed. Merck

4.   Marchant, T., Mushi, A.K., Nathan, R., Mukasa, O., Abdulla, S., Lengeler, C. and Armstrong Schellenberg, J.R.M. (2004). Planning a family: Priorities and Concerns in Rural Tanzania. *African Journal of Reproductive Health.* 8 (2): 111-123.

5.   Mturi, A.J. (2003). Parents' Attitudes to Adolescent Sexual Behaviour in Lesotho. *African Journal of Reproductive Health.* 7(2), pp. 25-33.

6.   Otoide, V. (2004). Targeting Adolescents for Family Planning and Post Abortion Care. *Tropical Journal of Obstetrics and Gynaecology.* 21(1), pp. 65-68.

7.   Plummer, M.L., Wight, D., Wamoyi, J., Nyalali, K., Ingall, T., Mshana, G., Shigongo, Z.S., Obasi, A.I. and Ross, D.A. (2006). Are schools a good setting for adolescent sexual health promotion in rural Africa? A qualitative assessment from Tanzania. *Health Education Research.* 22(4), pp. 483-499.

8.   Reeves, C., Whitaker, R., Parsonage, R.K., Robinson, C.A., Swale, K. and Bayley, L. (2006). Sexual Health Services and Education: Young people's experiences and preferences. *Health Education.* 65(4), pp. 368-379.

9.   Sunmola, A.M., Dipeolu, M., Babalola, S. and Adebayo, O.D. (2003). Reproductive knowledge, sexual behaviour and contraceptive use among adolescents in Niger State of Nigeria. *African Journal of Reproductive Health.* 7(1), pp. 37-48.

Chapter 16

CONTRACEPTION

Research has revealed that contraception may be seen as a preamble to sex in some cultures. A woman who has indulged in premarital sex may be seen in some cultures as spoiled and no longer pure and may be reviled, scorned and looked down upon by society as cheap and 'second hand' (Murira,2010). However, it is important that adolescents and young adults leaving high school should have information on the means available to prevent unwanted pregnancy. At this stage most young adults are ready to engage in sexual intercourse and may find it difficult to resist the urge to engage in sexual activity. Reckless sexual behaviours among youths have been associated with lack of sexual health information suggesting the need to educate youth to increase awareness of the risks of unprotected sexual activity (Wagbatsoma & Okojie, 2006).

Research has revealed that young women may know the sources of contraceptives and the names of some of the contraceptives, but they may have little knowledge about the contraceptives and how they could be used (Murira,2010).

While men are regarded as the decision makers and the family leaders, research has revealed that men in general are less informed about reproductive health than women(Lugalla et al.,2004;Cooper & Murira,2010). It is important that sexual health information is available to both young men and young women so that they behave responsibly, participate in prevention of pregnancy and refrain from unplanned unprotected sexual behaviours that result in pregnancy and teenage parenthood. Below are the commonly used contraceptive methods and the information that can benefit young people who may want to use contraception.

The Condom

The condom remains the most ideal method of contraception for its dual purpose of preventing pregnancy as well as preventing sexually transmitted diseases. There is no other method to date that has this dual function.

- The condom is ideal because it does not add additional hormonal load in the system of the user.
- It is easy to use.
- The condom is readily available in shops, chemists and local clinics.
- The condom does not need a doctor's prescription.
- It should be worn before a sexual act. There is also a female condom.
- After use one should wrap it in paper and dispose of it in a toilet.
- A condom should be used once for a single sexual act.
- Condoms must be kept away from the sun.

Research in Sub-Saharan Africa however suggests that men may perceive their partners' requests for condom use as evidence of female infidelity (Plummer et al.,2006). Women may therefore not insist on their men using the condom . In a survey of opinions of African men about the use of a condom. Cooper and Murira, (2010) found that men had very strong attitudes against the use of the condom which was likened to eating a sweet in its wrappers and also reported as reducing sensitivity and being a nuisance thus therefore suggesting that unless such attitudes change in some cultures, the use of the condom may not rise quickly. The teacher should inform the school leavers and college students on prevention of sexual infections and unwanted pregnancies through the use of a condom.

The Pill

The pill is in two types, the combined pill and the progesterone only pill.

- The individual potential user must consult with the source, the clinic, GP or chemist for a suitable pill according to one's health.
- One has to remember to take the pill every day preferably at the same time of the day to keep the levels of the chemical high in the blood.
- In the event of forgetting to take the pill but indulging in sexual activity, one has to take the **Morning after pill** that must be taken within forty-eight hours of sexual activity. This emergency contraception is

unfortunately least advertised and not readily available to would be users. Knowledge of emergency contraception has been found to be poor (Haggai,2003) and yet there is a need for awareness of this service.

- The pill affects the normal menstrual cycle in different ways in individual users.
- The combined pill may increase the menstrual flow while the progesterone only pill may cause scanty irregular flow or temporary cessation of menses.

Research shows that young people do not readily access contraceptive outlets for the pill, are not familiar with the use of the pill and their use is erratic (Ajayi et al.,1991; Amazigo, 1997; Marchant et al.,2004; Murira et al.,2010)

Implants

Implants are inserted under the skin by health personnel.

- Implants have similar action to the progesterone only pill. They are long acting but can be easily removed when one no longer wants them or is planning to fall pregnant (Aisien et al.,2004).

Intra-uterine Devices

Intra-uterine devices are available but these too must be inserted inside the uterus by a health specialist.

- They are suitable for an individual who has regular sexual contact.
- Intra-uterine devices have threads that a woman must feel when she washes to ensure that the device is in place.
- Both partners must observe very high standards of hygiene to prevent infection.

Foams

Young people may want to use foams and jellies which are instant contraceptives and whose action lasts through one sexual act.

There is no real reason for young people to carry an unwanted pregnancy. It is important that young people are aware that they can access contraception from the clinic, the chemist or to the GP's if they feel that they want to be sexually active.

Contraceptive programmes however continuously seek suitable methods and messages that persuade adolescents and young adults to develop positive attitudes towards premarital contraceptive use (Sunmola et al, 2003).

Health personnel are aware that young people prefer privacy when they seek contraceptive services. The presence of mature people in family planning centers may intimidate the young people who may feel that their reputation is under threat, (Murira et al., 2010). There are youth friendly clinics that can serve contraceptive needs of young people in private.

The pharmacist can assist in the provision of contraception in confidence. The teacher should keep in contact with health personnel for updates of health information and new health technologies available for adolescents.

Suggestions have been made that teachers get special training in sexual health education to increase young people's knowledge of sexual and reproductive health (Iyoke et al., 2006). Multiple interventions of teacher and peer education strategies have been found to improve knowledge, attitudes and self-efficacy in the sexual and reproductive health of students (Plummer et al.,2006; Ajuwon & Brieger, 2007).

There is however consensus among researchers that lack of standardised sexual health education in schools, and a lack of parental teaching and guidance of adolescents is largely to blame for careless sexual behaviours among young people(Mturi,2003;Wagbatsoma & Okojie, 2006; Ajuwon & Brieger, 2007; Babalola et al., 2007; Turnbull et al., 2008; Lema et al, 2008; Reeves et al,2006).

Essential medical examination

Young men and women should have a medical examination annually especially to exclude diseases that may emerge in adult life like high blood pressure and diabetes. Before starting a family, a medical check up is essential to exclude sexually transmitted diseases and have these treated thoroughly as they all can be passed onto the offspring resulting in poor pregnancy outcomes such as abortions and congenital abnormality of the newborn.

Before a young woman falls pregnant, she should undergo tests that exclude health problems, which may interfere with her health or impact on the pregnancy and successful pregnancy outcome.

Below are some essential medical tests that are necessary in young adults.

A Pelvic Examination

A sexually active young person must have a pelvic examination and a Pap smear which are essential tests to exclude cancers of the pelvic organs before falling pregnant.

Haemoglobin

Haemoglobin check ensures that a young adult approaches adulthood with healthy levels of haemoglobin in her blood. This is more so for young women intending to fall pregnant as pregnancy further lowers haemoglobin levels, causing anaemia, a situation that is detrimental to both the mother and the baby. It is advisable that abnormal levels of haemoglobin are corrected before one falls pregnant.

Blood pressure

Blood Pressure check is necessary to exclude essential hypertension, which may complicate adult life and pregnancy by affecting the mother's health as well predisposing the growing baby inside her to intra-uterine growth retardation, prematurity and related complications. The blood pressure may be elevated in a few children with underlying renal and liver pathology indicating a potential to develop high blood pressure as development continues.

Young adults have been observed to have a sudden spurt of high blood pressure at around the age of sixteen (Saha et al.,2008) . Some go on to develop essential hypertension from that age which goes unnoticed or the symptoms are taken lightly until one falls ill.

Breast Self-examination

Breast self examination is an essential skill in early diagnosis of tumours of the breast. Breast cancer is the second most common cancer in women. The most common cancer in women is cancer of the cervix. Every young woman should be able to do a breast self- examination to exclude lumps in the breast that could be suggestive of early cancer of the breast. Breast self examination is best done after a period in young people when the breast tissue is back to normal. Before a monthly period breast tissue is under the influence of female hormones which may alter the texture of the breast tissue resulting in false alarms and unnecessary anxiety.

Mature women (menopausal women) can examine their breasts at any time of the month. A young woman may do breast self-examination monthly after her menstrual cycle as described below.

Standing in front of a long mirror with a bare chest, look at the size of the breasts.

- The breasts should be symmetrical with the nipple in the centre.
- Lift hands up and again look at the size of the breasts.
- Inspect the skin of each breast. The skin should be smooth. If however there is change of skin colour, puckering or orange peel texture of the skin, report this observation to health personnel immediately.
- Now support one breast with the palm of one hand and start feeling for lumps in the breast tissue from the chest towards the nipple inspecting one small section of the breast at a time using flat fingers. Do not use the tips of the fingers. Repeat with the second breast.
- Health personnel can be invited to equip the young women with skills of breast self- examination. If one is not sure of what they are feeling or what they are observing, they should report to health personnel immediately.

Life sustaining medications

- Young adults taking anticoagulants, anti-asthmatic medications, anti-epileptic drugs and some antibiotics as well as those young adults with renal disease and heart disease should stay in contact with the physician for advice and adjustment of their medication. This is very important as some young adults feeling at the peak of their health may be tempted to ignore appointments with the doctor or stop taking medication completely.

- Adjustment of medication may be necessary when one changes a life style, increases or decreases activity, changes a diet, changes an environment, gains or looses weight, changes employment and prior to starting a family.

- Information on the impact of drugs used in controlling the medical conditions on fertility and pregnancy should be known so that one is aware of any impending risks and receives appropriate medical advice. The information helps in reaching informed decisions on planning for the size of family and the choice of appropriate family planning methods.

Exposure to metals and abnormal heat

Some cosmetics such as skin lightening creams and some face creams and lotions that clear blemishes and pimples may contain traces of lead. It is important to read labels and information on the levels of metals one is exposed to and the impact on other body systems like the renal system, and the cardiac and reproductive system.

Excessive heat

It is important that young people working in hot environments such as hot furnaces and kilns wear protective clothing supplied in such working environments. Heat alters scrotal temperatures and production of healthy sperms in adequate numbers.

Tight underwear generates heat which alters scrotal temperature. Young men should therefore opt for loose airy underclothes to keep that part of the body cool and maintain healthy scrotal temperatures.

Genetic Counselling

In some societies, children are considered an asset that every person must try to have. Genetic counselling is essential for young adults coming from families with conditions that run in the families like haemophilia, albinism and any congenital abnormalities in their families so that they have access to correct and relevant information that enables informed decision-making. The high school or college student should access this information as the future prospective parents.

Vaccination

Young people of ages 11-13 must have HBV vaccine that prevents cancer of the cervix. Young girls of age 15 years should have Rubella vaccine to prevent conditions that predispose the unborn baby to risk of abnormality due to exposure to rubella viral infection.

Nutritional Diseases

The importance of a good nutrition throughout the life span cannot be overemphasized. The stage of adolescence marks the beginning of the most active stage of development in life. While all parts of the body are striving to develop to their maximum, the young person is also reaching a stage where life's responsibilities demand of her/his energies to manage the multitudes of tasks demanded by adult life.

The young adult must be fit to meet the physical challenges of adult life as he/she breaks off from the care and protection of parents, from being a dependent, to being independent. Nutritionally related conditions such as anaemia and metabolic conditions such as diabetes are known to affect young people. An individual who is diagnosed of these conditions in late adolescence should immediately adhere to medical advice they get from health professionals. Low body weight at adolescence may be a disadvantage when one considers the physical demands ahead for instance in physical work that enables one to work for a daily leaving. Low body weight in young female adolescents is a disadvantage as it is associated with inability to nurture a pregnancy successfully resulting in premature labour and low birth weight of the newborn.

Preconception Education

Teenagers and young adults may fall pregnant as soon as they attain puberty or soon after puberty without access to pre-conception education. It is ideal that young adults leave high schools equipped with relevant information for the next stage in their development along the lifeline. Many young women meet with health personnel after they are already pregnant. Many young women go through the physiological transition from adolescence to women without the necessary prior knowledge and awareness of risks they are automatically exposed to in the new phase. Most young people do not associate their sexual behaviours with health problems such as sexually transmitted diseases including /HIV/AIDS and both male and female infertility.

It is advisable for young people to have health tests done and to acquire the relevant contraceptive protection before having sexual contact to protect themselves against preventable sexual and reproductive risks.

Some young people may have anxieties about securing a successful relationship. These anxieties should take into consideration the risk associated with unprotected sexual behaviours. Culture helps people to calculate risks and their consequences (Lupton, 1999).

The teacher has a role to understand the culture of the community in which he/she works in order to assist the learners to understand health risks. What may be deemed as a risk by professionals or by one culture may be viewed differently in another culture. Differences in perception affect how knowledge and understanding about risk may be developed in any particular group. It is therefore important that teachers emphasize the concept of sexual and reproductive risk to young people and the need for adolescents in any given culture to take appropriate preventive action against sexual and reproductive risk to their health.

Research reports on the limitations of schools in providing effective sexual health education that motivates young people to use contraception, as compared to health education provided for in health services that are specific in their approach to sexual education. It is desirable that school based health programmes be standardized, and specific to provide clear messages to young people (Aggleton, 1989; Abraham & Sheeran,1993; Wight et al., 2002). This is suggesting that school health programmes should not just be composed of biology of the reproductive system but useful life skills such as contraception.

A standardised school health curriculum ensures that all schools have access to evidence-based sexual health education to prevent misinformation or deprivation of some groups of children (Reeves et al., 2006). Lack of adolescent sexual health education exposes young people to sexual and reproductive complications that impact negatively on the health status of young women, increasing the risk of morbidity and mortality (Schulz et al., 2000).

Fig.1 Factors influencing teenage pregnancy (Murira,2010)

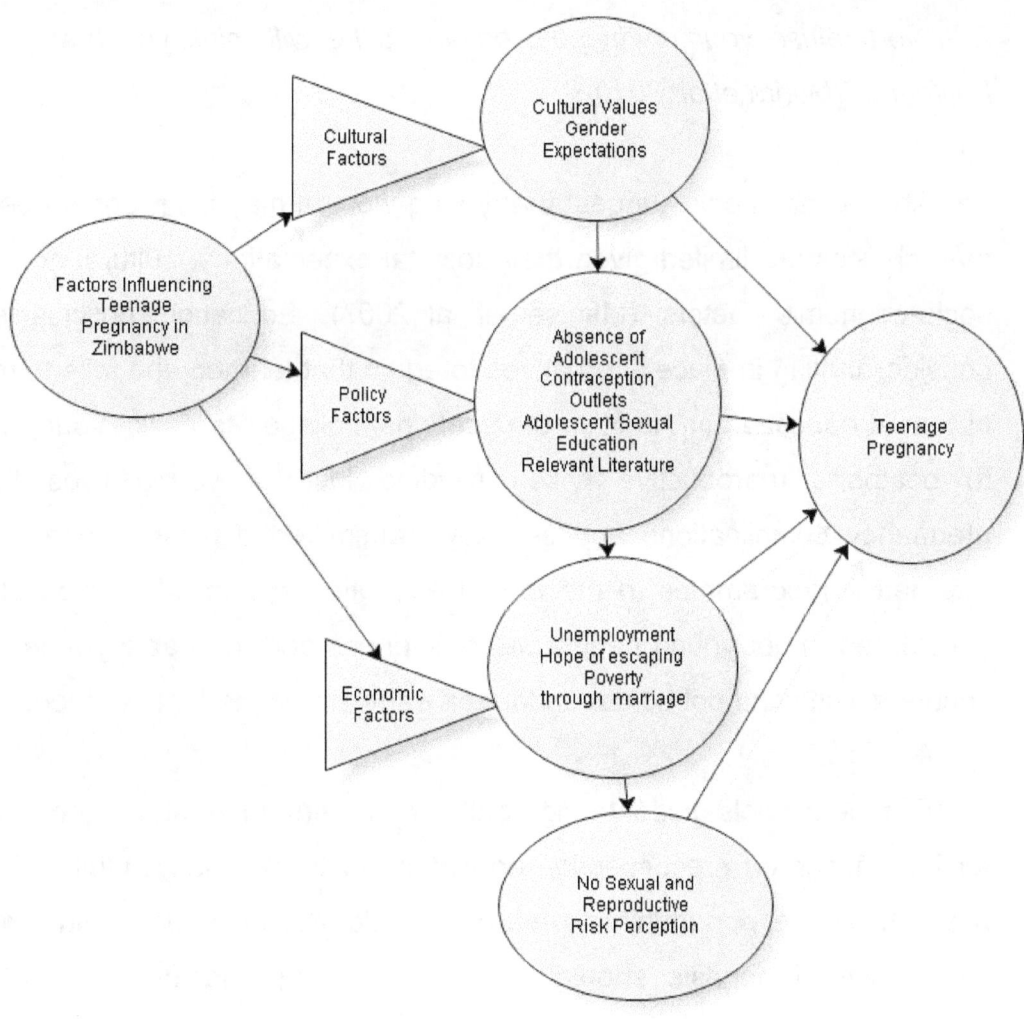

Research has revealed that young women's behaviour may be triggered by anxiety to safeguard their future.

 M.'When you no longer go to school what else is there to do? You might as well get a man and be married."

P."When you have a boyfriend and you refuse his advances he will leave you for another girl. If you want to be married the surest way is to fall pregnant."

Z."If you refuse your boyfriend's advances he will think you have another boyfriend."(Murira et al.,2010)

The above statements suggest that young women may fall pregnant because their choices are limited given their societal expectations, cultural norms and socio-economic factors (Madise et al.,2007). Education policies should consider putting in place alternatives to equip that learner who fails to make it in formal education in the form of vocational colleges to assist young people to postpone reproductive risks including loss of young lives through pregnancy complications and sexually transmitted diseases such as HIV. Alternative programmes to the formal education system should be strongly considered to get young people out of idleness and to enable young girls to secure a living and not be dependant on early marriages for livelihood.

At the time schools guide young adults on careers, there should be provision for information on preconception education for those young adults who may never have the opportunity to learn this information before falling into the family way. Emphasis should be on identifying and utilisation of local resources and working as a team with other disciplines and professionals to provide essential quality education that guides the young and future community and population leaders.

References
1. Abraham,C; Sheeran,P In search of a psychology of safer- sex promotion; beyond beliefs and text, *Health Education Research: Theory and Practice,*1993; 8: 245-54
2. Aggleton,P. HIV/AIDS Education in schools; constraints and possibilities, *Health Education Journal*, 1989; 48:167-71

3. Airhihenbuwa C.O; DeWitt Webster, J. Culture and African contexts of HIV/AIDS prevention, care and support. *Journal of Social Aspects of HIV/AIDS Research Alliance,*2004;1(1): 4-13

4. Aisien,A.O; Imade,G.E; Sagay,A.S et al., Safety, Efficacy and Acceptability of Norplant Implants in Jos, Northern Nigeria. *Tropical Journal of Obstetrics and Gynaecology,* 2004;21 (2): 42-49

5. Ajayi,A.A;Marangu,L.T;Miller,J et al., Adolescent sexuality in Kenya: A survey of knowledge, perceptions, and practices. *Studies in Family Planning* ,1991;22 (4): 205-216

6. Ajzen,I; Fishbein,M)*Understanding attitudes and predicting social behaviour.* Englewood Cliffs,1980. NJ: Prentice Hall

7. Ajuwon,A.J; Brieger,W.R. Evaluation of a school-based Reproductive Health Education programme in rural South Western, Nigeria. *African Journal of Reproductive Health,* 2007;11(2):47-59

8. Amazigo, U; Silva,N; Kaufman,J. et al., Sexual activity and contraceptive knowledge and use among in-school adolescence in Nigeria. *International Family Planning Perspective,* 1997;23(1): 215-220

9. Babalola,S; Tambashe, B.O; Vondrasek, C. Parental factors and sexual risk-taking among young people in Cote d'Ivoire. *African Journal of Reproductive Health.* 2005;9(1):123-128

10. Bankole,A; Biddlecom,A;Guiella,G. et al., Sexual Behaviour, Knowledge and Information Sources of Very Young Adolescents in Four Sub-Saharan African Countries. *African Journal of Reproductive Health,* 2007; 11 (3) : 99-105

11. Cooper,RG and Murira, N. Attitudes,Behaviours and Mechanics of male condom application: some considerations. The HIV/AIDS Newsletter,2010 Vol.3 No.1 pp2-3

12. Haggai,D. Emergency Contraception: A global Overview of Knowledge, Attitudes and Practices Among Providers. *Tropical Journal of Obstetrics and Gynaecology,* 2003; 20 (2): 56-65

13. Iyoke,C.A; Onah,H.E; Onwasigwe,C.N. Teachers' Attitude is not an impediment to Adolescent Sexuality Education in Enugu, Nigeria. *African Journal of Reproductive Health,* 2006; 10 (1): 81-90

14. Kankasa,C; Siwale,M; Kasolo F et al., Socioeconomic and reproductive factors associated with condom use within and outside of marriage among urban pregnant women in Zambia. African Journal of Reproductive Health, 2005; 9 (3):128-136

15. Keele,J.J; Forste,R; Flake,D,F. Hearing Native Voices: contraceptive use in Matemwe village, East Africa. *African Journal of Reproductive Health,* 2005;9 (1): 45-49

16. Lema, L.A., Katapa, R.S. and Musa, A.S. (2008). Knowledge of HIV/AIDS and sexual behaviour among youths in Kibaha District, Tanzania. *Tanzania Journal of Health Research.* 10(2), pp. 79-83.

17. Lupton, D. *RISK.* Routledge,1999. London and New York

18. Macintyre,S; McKay,L; Ellaway,A. Lay concepts of the relative importance of different influences on health; are there major socio-demographic variations? *Health Education Research Theory and Practice,* 2006; 21 (5):731-736

19. MacLachlan, M. *Culture and Health.* A Critical Perspective towards Global Health. 2nd Ed. John Wiley & Sons Ltd. 2006.Chichester.

20. Madise,N; Zulu,E; Ciera,J. Is poverty a driver for Risky Sexual Behaviour? Evidence from National Surveys of Adolescents in four African Countries. *African Journal of Reproductive Health,* 2007; 11(3): 83-98

21. Maria, W. (2006). Sexual Behaviour, Knowledge and Awareness of Related Reproductive Health Issues among Single Youth in Ethiopia. *African Journal of Reproductive Health.* 10(3), pp. 45-50.

22. Marchant,T; Mushi,AK; Nathan,R et alPlanning a family: Priorities and Concerns in Rural Tanzania. *African Journal of Reproductive Health,* 2004; 8 (2): 35-39

23. Murira,N; (2010) Communicating Sexual and Reproductive Health messages. Birmingham City University, Centre for Health and Social Care Research.

24. Mturi, A.J. Parents' Attitudes to Adolescent Sexual Behaviour in Lesotho. *African Journal of Reproductive Health,* 2003; 7 (2): 25-33

25. Otoide, V. Targeting Adolescents for Family Planning and Post Abortion Care. *Tropical Journal of Obstetrics and Gynaecology*, 2004; 21: (1): 65-68

26. Plummer, M.L; Wight, D.Wamoyi, J et al., Are schools a good setting for adolescent sexual health promotion in rural Africa? A qualitative assessment from Tanzania. *Health Education Research*, 2006; 22 (4): 483-499

27. Reeves, C; Whitaker,R; Parsonage R.K. et al., Sexual Health Services and Education: Young people's experiences and preferences. *Health Education*, 2006; 65 (4): 368-379

28. Saha, I; Paul, B; Dasgupta, A. Short communication: Prevalence of hypertension and variation of blood pressure with age among adolescents in Chetla, India. *Tanzania Journal of health Research*, 2008; 10 (2):108-111

29. Schulz, A.J; Krieger, J; Galea, S. Addressing social determinants of Health: Community Based participatory approaches to research and practice. *Health Education and Behaviour,* 2002; 29(3): 287-295

30. Sunmola, A.M; Dipeolu, M.; Babalola, S et al., Reproductive knowledge, Sexual behaviour and Contraceptive use among adolescents in Niger State of Nigeria. African Journal of Reproductive Health, 2003; 7(1):37-48

31. Turnbull, T; Wersch, A. Van Schaik. A review of parental involvement in sex education: The role for effective communication in British families. *Health Education Journal,* 2008: 67 (3):182-195

32. Wagbatsoma, V.A; Okojie, O.H. Knowledge of HIV/AIDS and Sexual Practices among Adolescents in Benin City Nigeria. *African Journal of Reproductive Health,* 2006; 10: (2) 76-83

33. Wight, D; Raab, G.M; Henderson, M et al., Limits of teacher delivered sex education: Interim behavioural outcomes from randomised trials. *BMJ*, 2002; 324:1430

Health Books by the same author

Mothers' Diary of Baby's Growth Milestones

Head to Toes (Everyday Health Book for Children)

Pregnancy, Labour, Self Care and Baby Care

Healthy Woman

Men's Health

About the Author

Nester Kadzviti Murira was educated to PhD level at Birmingham City University, UK, School of Health and Social Care Research. She has a Masters Degree in Medical Education from University of Dundee, Scotland, Centre for Medical Education. She has a B.Ed.Adult Education, and Diploma in Adult and Nursing Education from the University of Zimbabwe. She has a Diploma in Midwifery and General Nursing from Zimbabwe.

Nester has worked as a Health Care Training Consultant, a Lecturer in Reproductive Health, a Midwifery Tutor, a Research Midwife, a Maternity Home manager, and a Domiciliary Postnatal Services Care manager in Zimbabwe. Nester has worked in hospitals, care homes, and supported living under nursing agencies in several Primary Care Trusts in UK.

She is a published researcher and author of health books, children's books and contemporary subjects.

www.ingramcontent.com/pod-product-compliance
Lightning Source LLC
Chambersburg PA
CBHW080639180526
45168CB00008B/3227